The Private Self

THE PRIVATE SELF

Arnold H. Modell

HARVARD UNIVERSITY PRESS

Cambridge, Massachusetts
London, England
1993

Library of Congress Cataloging-in-Publication Data

Modell, Arnold H., 1924–
      The private self / Arnold H. Modell.
          p.   cm.
      Includes bibliographical references and index.
      ISBN 0–674–70752–4 (acid-free paper)
      1. Self-perception.   2. Social perception.   3. Self.   I. Title.
BF697.5.S43M63   1993
155'.2—dc20   93–14974
                                                                                        CIP

FOR ELLEN

Acknowledgments

In 1991 by a stroke of good fortune I was invited by Susan Borden, a trustee of the Neurosciences Institute, to join a study group of psychoanalysts and neuroscientists to explore the interface of neurobiology and psychoanalysis. I was privileged to meet with Gerald Edelman and his colleagues to discuss his theory of Neural Darwinism. It is as a result of these meetings that I developed the idea of applying the concept of biological value to the theory of the private self. The outline for this book had already been formed, but this first-hand encounter with Edelman's biological theory of consciousness proved serendipitous.

Gerald Edelman and his associates Giulio Tononi and Karl Friston, in the Department of Neurobiology of the Scripps Research Institute, read the manuscript and offered very valuable suggestions concerning its structure. The responsibility for this final version is, of course, my own.

I am grateful to my friend and colleague Donald Gerard, who also read the manuscript and advised me about some of the difficulties a reader might encounter.

Contents

The Private Self

Introduction

Some people would argue that a cobbler should stick to his last and not attempt to do that which is above his station. They would claim that a psychoanalyst should stick to what he knows best, which is clinical psychoanalysis, and leave philosophy and neurobiology to experts in those fields. This advice can be followed if the subject being investigated lies nearly entirely within the borders of psychoanalysis, such as the concept of the id or of the superego. The topic of the self, however, which is of recent clinical interest to psychoanalysts, has been explored by philosophers for at least two millennia. My critics may respond that the self of the philosopher is not the self the psychoanalyst observes in his or her daily work, and that therefore the psychoanalyst can safely ignore the philosopher's self. But the concept of a self cannot possibly be derived entirely from clinical observation, for whether or not we are aware of their influence, philosophers have shaped certain assumptions regarding the self that are part of our modern sensibility.

There is an additional reason the contributions of philosophers cannot be ignored in this book: one must take into account the unavoidable epistemological dilemma posed by an outside observer's observing the private self. I suspect that because of this dilemma, Freud, instead of embracing a phenomenology of self and basing his theories on the subjective experiences of the self, chose a more "scientific" path describing an "ego," a mental apparatus. How can the individual's private experience of the self be treated as a scientific "objective reality" by other persons? This is the problem that philosophers have been attempting to solve ever since Descartes separated the mind from things in the world. Although there appears to be no solution, the view I find most congenial is the position taken by William James: the experience of self is a fundamental reality which cannot be transposed or reduced into something else that is more "objective."

Since I am not a philosopher and have had no formal training in philosophy, this book is not in any sense a contribution to philosophy. But no consideration of the self can afford to ignore the discussion that William James set forth in his *Principles of Psychology;* I review his contributions in Chapter 1. I have also found the work of a contemporary philosopher, John Searle, to be particularly relevant to the problem of the mind and the brain (see Chapter 6).

In my previous book, *Other Times, Other Realities,* I was influenced by Gerald Edelman's *Neural Darwinism,* especially his theory of memory as recategorization. This theory fitted in very well with my psychoanalytic observations of the therapeutic process. In a subsequent book, *The Remembered Present,* Edelman proposed a neurobiological theory of consciousness and the self in an evolutionary context. He suggested that as a higher order of consciousness evolved, awareness of the self conferred on the individual a distinct adaptive advantage, permitting the organism to develop a coherent internal model of past, present, and future, and thus enabling it to be free of the tyranny of ongoing events in present time. In human beings and perhaps in other highly intelligent mammals, the brain maps not only significant features in the external world but also the individual's inner, psychological state. We describe the latter as "consciousness of self." Edelman's theory suggests that, in a deep biological sense, the private self enables the individual to become more psychologically autonomous.

In *Psychoanalysis in a New Context* and *Other Times, Other Realities,* I suggested that paradox is an intrinsic quality of the human mind. In *The Private Self* I shall claim that in order to understand the nature of the self, we must recognize its fundamentally paradoxical nature. The self endures through time as a sense of identity, yet consciousness of self is always changing. The self derives its sense of coherence and continuity from within, yet at the same time depends on the appraisals of others, who can either support or disrupt the self's continuity. The self is paradoxical: it is an enduring structure and at the same time nearly coterminus with an ever-changing consciousness. Furthermore, the private self supports a relative self-sufficiency, whereas from another perspective the self is not at all autonomous but can be seen as vulnerable in its dependence upon others for a sense of coherence and continuity.

The ability to accept paradox, I believe, results in a mind set that enables one to tolerate inconsistency and contradiction without forcing a premature closure. The willingness to accept paradox is probably a matter of temperament, and is associated with a capacity for play. I associate the acceptance of paradox with a certain intellectual openness and playfulness. Yet I recognize that such a mind set may not be congenial to readers who tend to think in dichotomies— who think that something must be either this or that, not this *and* that. Readers lacking a taste for paradox might find this book difficult to understand.

This dichotomous mind set has been characteristic of much of the notable literature concerning the self. To avoid appearing inconsistent and contradictory, most authors have viewed the self exclusively either as a psychic structure or as coterminus with consciousness. Freud avoided the term "self," preferring to describe the shadow of lost objects that falls upon the ego. Although one's sense of identity is more than the sum of one's identifications, the continuity of the self can be explained, in part, as a reflection of lasting identifications with formerly loved persons. William James, on the other hand, chose to describe the self not as a psychic structure but as an inner awareness of the ever-changing stream of consciousness.

In Chapter 1, where I attempt to survey these and other contributions to our thinking about the self, I have been obliged to unpack the paradox of structure and consciousness by presenting these views separately. My lengthy opening chapter may present problems for some readers because it is textually "dense," and because my own ideas concerning the private self do not appear until Chapters 2 and 3.

In Chapter 2, I marshal convergent observations from psychoanalysis, infant research, and neurobiology that support the concept of a private self. I then review various concepts of the social self, such as Heinz Kohut's "selfobject" and the self as formulated by George Herbert Mead and by Erving Goffman.

In emphasizing the vital significance of the private self, I am striving to correct a current bias that views the self nearly exclusively as a social self. Many contemporary authors have exaggerated the significance of this social aspect of the self, minimizing or neglecting the self's capacity to "bootstrap" itself from within. As many life experiences attest, there are individuals who have been able to "create" themselves and maintain a sense of continuity and coherence despite extremely traumatic childhoods. It seems to me that the oft-repeated assertion of self psychologists—namely, that the self's need for affirming selfobjects is equivalent to the organism's need for oxygen—is a misleading statement. This overemphasis on the social self, to the relative neglect of the private self, is also illustrated by social psychologists' claim that the self acquires meaning not from within but through the acquisition of cultural narratives.

Researchers who emphasize the social self at the expense of the private self also tend to view the self as disembodied—that is, they claim that one can consider the self apart from biology. I firmly believe, however, that the psychology of the self is rooted in biology; to think otherwise is a profound error.

William James in philosophy and Donald Winnicott in psychoanalysis are among the few authors who have recognized the paradox of the self. James, throughout his life, struggled with the fact that the concept of self encompasses both a stable sense of identity and a transient consciousness. He was unable to reconcile how a momentary state of consciousness could connect with the stored memories of previous selves and create the unity that we experience as identity. There is also no doubt that James viewed the self as embodied, for in his panoramic account of the self, James begins with the declaration that the body is the innermost part of the material self.

My concept of the private self owes a great deal to Winnicott's notion of the "true" self. Winnicott believed that the true self cannot be thought of as anything other than a manifestation of the psyche-soma. And Winnicott repeatedly advised his readers of the importance of accepting paradox. In Chapter 5, I discuss the implications of one such Winnicottian paradox: that, initially, the capacity for solitude requires the mother's presence.

Most experienced clinicians would not question the existence of a private self, for in their daily work they can observe the way in which patients protect the private self from intrusion. Psychopathology illustrates the vulnerability of the private self, yet pathology only exaggerates that which is present in all of us. It is true that we are dependent upon the affirmation of others for our sense of identity, but it is equally true that others can disrupt our continuity of self. The private self is altered when in public space. In Chapter 3, I present a detailed clinical vignette of a patient who feared that other people could disrupt the continuity and coherence of her self.

Some readers may question the absence of additional detailed case material. For reasons of confidentiality, however, I have been unable to use case histories to illustrate my theoretical positions. Readers will have to accept, as a matter of trust, that what I write is always informed by my experience as a practicing psychoanalyst.

Researchers who work with infants support the idea of a private self. They have observed that infants are aware of their separateness from their mothers. When infants are posited as separate beings, certain autonomous functions of the self can be inferred. The infant regulates periods of engagement and disengagement with its mother, so that periods of disengagement have a place of equal importance. At times of disengagement, the infant experiences a sense of "being fueled from within." These observations suggest that pleasure can be generated in states of nonrelatedness, in which the child is free to follow its own interests. Winnicott described this free activity as the infant's "spontaneous gesture." The child takes obvious joy in mastery.

Edelman's neurobiological theory likewise gives support to the idea of a private self. In addition to the evolutionary advantage mentioned above, the experience of self enables the individual to model future actions by matching value-laden memories of past events with current perceptions. From a biological perspective, consciousness of self enables one to be relatively autonomous from environmental inputs. These ideas are discussed in Chapter 2.

In Chapter 4, I investigate the psychology of merging and separateness. Here I have been guided by Hegel's parable of the master/slave relationship, which formulates the dialectics of self and other in relation to the asymmetry of power and desire. I also discuss the idea that a multileveled consciousness provides the self with a measure of freedom.

The private self can also be described as the locus of personal values and passionate interests. In Chapter 5, I show how such passionate interests can sustain one in states of solitude. I also discuss Winnicott's paradox, mentioned above: that the capacity for solitude initially requires the mother's presence. In adult life, this paradoxical aspect of solitude can be seen in the relationships of creative individuals to their muse. I explore several of these relationships by referring to biographical studies.

When I began to write this book, I viewed the paradox of the self as the organizing principle. As the work progressed, however, I developed additional aims and concerns. This has affected the book's design: the last three chapters (6, 7, and 8) have a focus that is somewhat different from that of the preceding ones. Chapters 6–8 contain a discussion of the creation of personal or private meaning—an argument for the *biological* agency of the self. In Chapter 6, I discuss the evidence for the existence of unconscious structures of the self, and the relation between those structures and the generation of meaning. The inability to create new meanings I view as a psychic catastrophe often termed a "black hole." In Chapters 6–8 I attempt to connect the agency of the self with the creation of new meanings, claiming that the coherence and continuity of the self are augmented when the self extends its agency through the creation of new meanings. My ideas receive a certain support from Edelman's theory of "biological value," which illuminates the problem of the emergent motives of the self. I view the idea of biological value as a potential replacement for the concept of instinct (see Chapter 8). This is not to suggest a simple-minded reduction of psychoanalytic concepts to those of neurobiology; such a replacement would be impossible. But certain psychoanalytic concepts such as instinct are, as Freud recognized, on the border between physiology and psychology and as such must be congruent with contemporary neuroscience.

In addition to urging readers to recognize the paradoxical nature of the self, I therefore emphasize that *the self is embodied. Within the self there is a unity of the psyche-soma: brain and mind are a seamless web.*

1

Thinking about the Self: Structure and Consciousness

> Personality implies the incessant presence of two elements, an objective person, known by a passing subjective thought and recognized as continuing in time.
> WILLIAM JAMES, *Principles of Psychology*, vol. 2

Let us now survey the contributions of those who view the self as a psychic structure, and contrast their ideas with those of other authors who equate the self with consciousness. In this chapter the paradox of structure and consciousness will be, at least temporarily, unpacked. A concurrent theme will be the philosophical dilemma of describing the private experience of self from the perspective of an outside observer.

Let's first examine the self as a psychic structure, and then consider the phenomenology of the self—that is, the self as an aspect of consciousness. Freud and William James will serve as exemplars. Although we'll be looking at the two wings of the paradox separately, we should keep in mind that a viable theory of the self must encompass the interrelationship between unconscious process and conscious experience.

Consciousness of one's self—that is to say, self consciousness—is a constantly changing experience. This is the self that has been described by philosophers from Saint Augustine to William James who have observed themselves by means of introspection. William James's stream of consciousness *is* the self. Yet there is another aspect of the self that we trust will remain relatively unchanged—that is, our identity. So that despite the flux of experience, there is a core of the self that remains the same. This is to claim not an absolute sameness but a recognizable sameness, an ability to recover one's identity despite whatever happens to one.[1] Some researchers think this restorative quality of identity is so vital that it represents a biological principle analogous to homeostasis.[2]

Although Freud avoided the term "self" *(selbst)*,[3] the concept of self is implicit in his structural theory of the ego. In his opinion, a purely phenomenological, subjective account of the self experience was unscientific, when compared to the objective concept "ego." Freud was confronted with the fundamental epistemological dilemma concerning the self. It is a dilemma that philosophy has yet to resolve. How does one transpose an individual's private and unique experience of his or her own self into the conceptual system of an external scientific observer bent on "objectifying" that experience? To objectify the experience of self is to place it within a generalized impersonal schema such as an ego, which then violates the uniqueness of the self.

Philosophers of the self have for the most part followed William James in equating the self with consciousness, whereas psychoanalysts, following Freud, have focused on the structural and unchanging aspects of the self. Exceptions are Paul Federn and, more recently, Heinz Kohut.

There is perhaps a third school of thought, which doubts the existence of the self. The evanescence of the consciousness of self has led some philosophers, psychiatrists, and psychoanalysts to doubt whether the self actually exists. In philosophy, David Hume is considered the principal spokesman for this skeptical position. From a psychoanalytic perspective (as William Grossman says), if the self depends on one's view of oneself, the self may be only a "fantasy." Hume describes the mutability of the experience of self as follows: "Nor is there any single power of the soul which remains unalterably the same, perhaps for one moment. The mind is a kind of theatre, where several perceptions successively make their appearance; pass, repass, glide away, and mingle in an infinite variety of postures and situations. There is properly no *simplicity* in it at one time, nor *identity in different [times], whatever natural propensity we may have to imagine that simplicity and identity.*"[4]

A contemporary philosopher, Robert Nozick,[5] holds the opposite view—that at least an illusion of an unchanging identity persists over time—and he illustrates this idea with the following thought experiment. Imagine that your brain has been transplanted into another person's body, and that the other person's brain has been transplanted into your body. Upon which body would you choose to have pain inflicted? Your answer would no doubt be: your former body, in which the other person's brain now resides. For most of us imagine that the self, which we selfishly protect, resides in our brain, with its unique and particular store of memories. We also imagine that our sense of self, our identity, will continue no matter where it is transplanted, provided that our brain remains intact.

There is clinical evidence that loss of the sense of continuity of the self is a psychic catastrophe. Winnicott believed that when the maternal environment fails to provide the infant with a sense of continuity of being, the child can develop a sense of unbearable annihilation anxiety.[6] Schizophrenic patients were the first to teach us about this phenomenon. Such patients described their fear of having no self, of being swallowed up in another person's identity. The fear that one's sense of identity can be destroyed in an instant is not felt only by schizophrenics. Many other people also experience their identity as something that is extremely fragile and vulnerable. For some, their sense of a continuity of being is held hostage to the response of another person. As one of my patients described it, she felt as if her sense of self could be completely sucked out and obliterated by others. As a child, she had had the fantasy that an octopus used its tentacles to suck out the contents of its victims, and she believed that her sense of identity could be analogously sucked out by the other. Her sense of self was not threatened when she was alone, but she always felt vulnerable in the presence of others, especially if they were strangers.

For anyone who experiences annihilation anxiety, who fears that his or her sense of self is disintegrating, the existence of the self is not a matter for philosophical debate. The feeling that the self is becoming fragmented, transformed, or annihilated evokes the most terrible anxiety that anyone is likely to experience. The apprehension of a self that is continuous over time is thus not an illusion, as Hume would claim, but something that is essential to our existence.

As a counterpoise to the experience of a continuing self, consciousness of self is always changing in reaction to the affirming or negating responses of others. We need not turn to pathology to find illustrations of this: everyone's sense of self is modified in response to others. The self is inevitably altered in public space. This experience of self is not only dependent on the responses of others but is also affected by one's internal environment, such as changes in mood. Some people suffer rapid fluctuations of self esteem, veering from a sense of grandiose expansiveness to a feeling of constricted helplessness. Such reversals can occur almost instantaneously.

* * *

Although Freud avoided using the term "self," his theory of the "I" (ego) can be read as a theory of the self. He posited a self that is colored by its lasting identifications with others, as in his famous statement in "Mourning and Melancholia": "Thus the shadow of the object fell upon the ego."[7] But Freud also recognized that the ego is more than the sum of its identifications.

Freud's notion of the self is unlike that of William James (the self as the stream of the experience of consciousness), for Freud believed that a pure phenomenology of the self would elude scientific description. In his view, the structures of the ego are the result of identifications with loved persons, and identity is in turn derived from one's identifications. At the height of ego psychology in the 1950s, psychoanalysts had only a peripheral interest in the self as such, but they devoted some attention to the topic of ego identity. Erik Erikson, who coined the term "identity crisis," understood that one's identity is something that is both self created and bestowed upon the individual by the culture. For Erikson, the concept of identity lies on the border between psychology and sociology.[8] "*Identity formation* finally begins where the usefulness of identification ends," he declared. "It arises from the selective repudiation and mutual assimilation of childhood identifications, and their absorption in a new configuration, which, in turn, is dependent on the process by which a *society identifies the young individual.*"[9]

The self as consciousness was therefore largely ignored by psychoanalysts, except in the case of an original such as Paul Federn.[10] Not until the phenomenology of the self became the focus of Kohut's new "self psychology" did the self as consciousness receive proper attention. Kohut's self psychology is a radical departure from Freudian psychoanalysis in that it is based entirely on the patient's subjective experience. As such, it occupies a separate philosophical realm.

Although Kohut refers to psychic structures, structural concepts—which are abstractions remote from experience—receive little elaboration in his work. The two sides of the paradox—the structural continuity of the self and its discontinuity in consciousness—thus have been considered in tandem by very few researchers. An exception was William James, who, although he focused on the self as consciousness, was fully aware of the paradox of the self (continuity amid an ever-changing consciousness).

Freud avoided the pitfalls of "unscientific" subjectivity by conceptualizing the self as an objective structure, the ego. The term "ego," as used in psychoanalysis, is an abstraction, a mental "apparatus" defined by its functions. Freud, in *The Ego and the Id,* defined the ego as "a coherent organization of mental processes."[11] The difference between the objective ego and the subjective self can be illustrated by referring to the topic of anxiety: the self *experiences* anxiety, whereas the ego *responds* to a signal of unpleasure that is automatic and unconscious.[12] Anxiety can be considered either as an impersonal process impinging on the self or as a personal experience. (This point will be expanded in Chapters 6 and 7.) In this respect, the ego's use of signal anxiety is no different from other physiological responses the body employs to maintain homeostasis. Thus, the ego can be defined in accordance with its functions as if it were a bodily organ. But the continuity and coherence of the self also constitute a homeostatic function that is vital to the individual's psychological health. Generalizing in this fashion about the self confronts us with the same epistemological dilemma. As the philosopher Charles Taylor has stated:

> Here [in the problem of the objectification of the self] we see the origin of one of the great paradoxes of modern philosophy. The philosophy of disengagement and ob-

jectification has helped to create a picture of the human being, at its most extreme in certain forms of materialism, from which the last vestiges of subjectivity seem to have been expelled. It is a picture of the human being from a completely third-person perspective. The paradox is that this severe outlook is connected with, indeed, based on, according a central place to the first-person stance. This paradox has, of course, been much commented on by Heidegger, for instance, in his critique of subjectivism, and by Merleau-Ponty. Modern naturalism can never be the same once one sees this connection, as both these philosophers argue. But for those who haven't seen it, the problem of the "I" returns, like a repressed thought, as a seemingly insoluble puzzle.[13]

Since philosophy has found this problem intractable, we can hardly expect that psychoanalysis could come up with a definitive solution. But as some researchers have suggested,[14] Freud may have unwittingly contributed to solving the problem of the objectification of subjectivity.

Freud on Persons and Structure

Although Freud the scientist felt compelled to translate his observations of his patients' experiences into the abstraction of a mental apparatus, the humanist in him prevented him from doing so completely. Accordingly, he alternated between an anthropomorphic account of psychic structures, which treated these structures as if they themselves were persons, and a very different account in which the formation of psychic structures was seen as an impersonal process based on the transformation of instinctual energy.[15] In his anthropomorphic account Freud preserved the experiential aspect of the self,[16] whereas in his impersonal account he adhered to the requirements of objective science. In the first instance, Freud described the ego and the superego as if they were people—a child and its parents: the superego is at times punitive toward the ego, whereas at other times it is loving and protective. As Freud said in "Group Psychology and the Analysis of the Ego": "Let us reflect that the ego now enters into the relation of an object to the ego ideal which has been developed out of it, and that all the interplay between an external object and the ego as a whole, with which our study of the neuroses has made us acquainted, may possibly be repeated upon this new scene of action within the ego."[17] And in "An Outline of Psychoanalysis," he said: "A portion of the external world has, at least partially, been abandoned as an object and has instead, by identification, been taken into the ego and thus become an integral part of the internal world. *This new psychical agency continues to carry on the functions which have hitherto been performed by the people [the abandoned objects] in the external world: it observes the ego, gives it orders, judges it and threatens it with punishments, exactly like the parents whose place it has taken.*"[18] Freud believed that the superego could be loving and protective, as well as persecutory, in its relations with the ego: "The fear of death in melancholia only admits of one explanation: that the ego gives itself up because it feels itself hated and persecuted by the super-ego, instead of loved. To the ego, therefore, living means the same as being loved—being loved by the super-ego. The super-ego fulfills the same function of protecting and saving that was fulfilled in earlier days by the father, and later by Providence or Destiny."[19]

Within these anthropomorphic descriptions are interspersed more "scientific" accounts of the development of psychic structure. The following is typical: "The super-ego arises, as we know, from an identification with the father taken as a model. Every such identification is in the nature of a desexualization or even of a sublimation. It now seems as though when a transformation of this kind takes place, an instinctual defusion occurs at the same time."[20]

Researchers who have claimed that psychoanalysis is a positivistic science[21] have criticized Freud for not distinguishing the self from the ego.[22] Perhaps these critics did not fully recognize the philosophical dilemma with which Freud was confronted. Freud was not philosophically naive and could not have been unaware of the problems inherent in objectifying experience. More probably, Freud understood that the ambiguity between the objectified "I" and the experiencing "I" was not resolvable. Therefore, he depicted a personal self, in conjunction with an ego in the context of a mental apparatus. *He chose the strategy of shifting from one domain to the other.*

Freud's carefully sustained ambiguity regarding the domains of the personal and the impersonal was disrupted by James Strachey's English translation of Freud's works, which has become the subject of increasing criticism.[23] By creating a new vocabulary of Greek and Latin terms,[24] Strachey created the impression in the English-speaking world that psychoanalysis was a strictly scientific undertaking. For example, Strachey translated Freud's *Ich* "I" as "ego." Sometimes Freud's language was replaced by terms that were totally invented by Strachey, such as "cathexis" for *Besetzung*.[25]

When describing psychic structures as persons, Freud depicted two somewhat different outcomes. First, there may be a misidentification with the other person. This misidentification is usually unconscious; individuals behave as if they were the other person, without any awareness of the source of their behavior. In "Mourning and Melancholia," Freud observed that if an ambivalently loved object has been internalized and identified with the self, the individual misidentifies with that other person and, in a sense, becomes that other person. The self hatred, self accusations, and self depreciation of the melancholic refer not to the self but to someone else. Second, the gestalt of an entire *relationship* between the self and the object in the external world may be transposed into the self.

We know that this phenomenon of the self misidentifying itself is by no means limited to depression. It is a widespread method by which one can preserve a belief in the "goodness" of the object by assimilating into one's self the "bad" or unwanted attributes of the other person. One can continue to love the "bad" parent, whose "badness" is thus magically ingested and disposed of. It is as if the child were saying, "I would rather be bad in order to preserve the illusion of the power, effectiveness, and goodness of my parent."

We must also allow for the fact that what is internalized into the self may also contain elements of the parent's unconscious attitudes regarding the child. Thus, the sense of self may be, in part, formed through the *parents'* unconscious attitudes toward themselves and their own internalized parental objects. In this fashion, a certain family culture is preserved.[26] A mother, for example, may unconsciously identify her son with her own father and project onto the son a constellation of thoughts and feelings originally experienced in relation to her father; or the mother may unconsciously identify the child with aspects of her hated or beloved self; and so forth. In one instance, the child is the active agent in its attempt to assimilate the parent's "badness" so as to preserve a belief in the parent's "goodness." In the other instance, the child is the passive recipient of the parent's unconscious projections. The nature of these unconscious identifications of the self is therefore colored not only by experience but by the fantasies of both child and parent.

Fairbairn's Notion of Endopsychic Structures

Freud's observation that a *relationship* between the self and the object can be transposed from the external world into the self became the starting point for W. R. D. Fairbairn's theory of endopsychic structures.[27] This theory of the self differed from that of Freud in many significant respects. Fairbairn rejected Freud's instinct theory and believed instead that the self is energized by internal relations with exciting, frustrating, and persecuting objects. This internal dynamic, he believed, makes a theory of instinct unnecessary. Libido,[28] he maintained, is primarily object seeking and not pleasure seeking. An instinct theory is superfluous, because the energy of the impulse is contained in the psychic structures. His formula "energy = structure" was evidently influenced by Einstein's discoveries. Fairbairn thought that psychic structures were equivalent to relations with internalized persons.

Freud's concept of erotogenic zones, if these are conceived as something apart from object relationships, made no sense to Fairbairn. "The conception of fundamental erotogenic zones constitutes an unsatisfactory basis for any theory of libidinal development because it is based on a failure to recognize that the function of libidinal pleasure is essentially to provide a sign-post to the object. 'Impulses' cannot be considered apart from the endopsychic structures which they energize and the object-relationships which they enable these structures to establish; and equally 'instincts' cannot profitably be considered as anything more than forms of energy which constitute the dynamic of such endopsychic structures."[29]

I suspect that all major psychological discoveries appear first as an intuition derived from self observation, which is then extended to others as a universal principle. There is a long tradition for such self observation, ranging from Saint Augustine to Freud. A similar piece of self observation led to Fairbairn's concept of exciting and persecutory objects within the self. John Sutherland, in his account of Fairbairn's life and work, demonstrates the connection between specific traumatic events in Fairbairn's childhood and the content of his theory.[30] Sutherland tells of a particular episode in which Fairbairn, as a boy, saw some bloodstained menstrual pads in a pail and questioned his mother about them, whereupon she flew into a rage.[31] Fairbairn had a marked sexual curiosity, which, in the context of his relationship with his mother, he experienced as both exciting and forbidden. Just as Freud viewed his own Oedipus complex as universal, Fairbairn elevated this self observation to the status of a universal theory of psychic structures, expressed as sexually exciting and prohibiting internalized objects. The details of this are revealed in Fairbairn's diagram of psychic structures, in which he portrayed a central ego and a libidinal ego with corresponding rejecting and exciting internal objects.[32] The important point is that here the structure of the self represents an internalization of a *relationship*.[33] Fairbairn viewed psychic structures as a record of traumatic interactions, whereas for Freud, these structures represented a mosaic of lost objects.

Fairbairn intended his theory of endopsychic structures to be a reply in his dialogue with Freud—his reply to "The Ego and the Id."[34] Unfortunately, he retained Strachey's language, referring to the "ego" rather than to the "I" or to the "self." He posited the existence of a central ego, distinct from the internalized objects with which it has relations. So Fairbairn's self, like the self of William James and (as we shall see) the self of George Herbert Mead, contains both a subject and an object. Fairbairn's theory, with its central

ego, libidinal ego, internal saboteur, and exciting and rejecting objects, is much more complex than Freud's tripartite
model. Fairbairn's central thesis—that the self consists of
internalized relationships—remains relevant for contemporary psychoanalytic theory, whereas the details of his
model of the self have been politely ignored.

Fairbairn believed that within a self that is initially uni-
tary and object-seeking, dissociative splits develop as a result of traumatic *interactions* between the child and its caretakers. For example, the nonacceptance of the child by its
caretakers may result in an analogous split within the central self, so that the child does not accept itself and becomes
dissociated from part of itself. Perhaps the clearest exposition of this theory is provided by Fairbairn, as rendered by
Sutherland: "[Fairbairn] regards the *developed* psyche as a
multiplicity of structures of two classes, ego structures and
internal objects. The latter are conceived of as introjected
and structured as representations of emotionally significant
aspects of persons upon whom the subject depended in early
life. The internal object is an endopsychic structure, other
than an ego structure, with which an ego structure has a relationship comparable to a relationship with a person in external reality."[35]

Fairbairn thus dealt with the self/ego dilemma via the totally explicit anthropomorphism of internalized object relations. He understood psychic structures to be representations
of the emotionally significant aspects of persons, thereby
avoiding the difficulty of trying to describe the personal self
in impersonal terms. But there is a logical problem here, because, strictly speaking, psychic structures can never be personal. Since they can never be directly experienced, we can
say only that they *generate* experience. (This issue is discussed in more detail in Chapter 6.)

Fairbairn believed that the self is a coherent, object-seeking entity from the beginning—a view that finds support in recent research on infants.[36] The fact that Fairbairn freed himself from Freud's impersonal theory of instinct also allowed him to view the self as a source of *personal* morality. In contrast, Freud's concept of the superego derived its strength from impersonal instinctual forces, although Freud acknowledged the influence of other sources such as parents and teachers. Fairbairn's "internal saboteur," with its automatic response of guilt, corresponds closely to Freud's superego. But then Fairbairn suggested that the superego operates at a higher level than does the internal saboteur.[37] He seemed to suggest that conscience and morality can be attributed to two different structures: one automatic and impersonal, and the other more self generative, representing more personal moral values. Fairbairn explained in a footnote that he retained the term "super-ego" to refer to an internal object that is accepted as "good" and which appears to function as an ego ideal (a higher level of organization than that of the internal saboteur).[38] Fairbairn further suggested that this "good" superego may serve as a defense against "bad" internal objects. Whatever we think of Fairbairn's formulation, he, more clearly than Freud, separated an ego ideal representing personal values from an instinctual superego, whereas Freud tended to confuse these two concepts.[39] (One must admit, though, that Fairbairn's terminology obscures this point.)

Let us digress for a moment in order to examine Freud's more impersonal concept of the superego. Freud, in speculating on the origin of the superego, relied on what he believed to be a Darwinian concept. (His misunderstanding of Darwinism will be discussed in Chapter 8.) He believed that the superego originated in the earliest history of the human race. In this regard he was influenced by Lamarck's theory of evolution. Freud attributed the development of the superego to a racial memory of the threat of punishment from the primordial father. In accordance with Haeckel's Law, which Freud accepted, the development of the individual recapitulates the trauma that the species encountered.[40] Freud continued to believe, for example, that the fear of castration, which characterizes the relation between the ego and superego, resulted from a racial memory of the murder of the father by the primal horde of sons, as described in "Totem and Taboo." Freud reiterates this belief in "The Ego and the Id": "The super-ego, according to our hypothesis, actually originated from the experiences that led to totemism."[41]

For Freud it was this impersonal instinct theory, interpreted in accordance with the biology of his time, that provided the foundation upon which notions of personal experience could be centered. But Freud did not completely ignore the development of a personal morality: he noted that superego formation also reflects the history of the individual. It was, he said, also influenced by "the earliest parental imagoes."[42]

The Limitations of Fairbairn's Theory

Fairbairn's vision of a self that is derived from interpersonal relationships is pivotal in the intellectual history of psychoanalysis. Yet although I've been drawn to Fairbairn's ideas since my first years in psychiatry, his theory still seems to me to be somewhat arid: it lacks a sense of psychic aliveness. Furthermore, it does not acknowledge the consciousness of a self in real time. Internalized object relations are structures that memorialize old struggles, and it is not clear how

Fairbairn's theory would translate memories into experience.

Otto Kernberg's theory of internalized object relations is an important addition to Fairbairn's concepts.[43] Kernberg proposed the significant idea that *affects are the organizers of internalized objects.* This, however, was a kind of hybrid theory combining Fairbairn's ideas with the instinct theory of classical ego psychology, which Fairbairn had rejected.

Internalized Relationships within the Self

All the unique characteristics of the relationship between child and parent may be recreated within the self. Thus, the self contains, within itself, both subject and object. The self is hated and loved, punished and protected, aroused and inhibited, inspired and negated. The behavior of the self toward itself mirrors in every conceivable way the experiences in which the self is an object to others.

Patients often reveal that a very specific pattern of interaction with a parent is recreated within the self. Someone whose mother was unable to soothe or comfort her when she was a child, for example, is unable to soothe or comfort herself as an adult. Patients whose mothers were careless, neglectful, and indifferent to them recreate the same attitude of carelessness and indifference toward themselves. If a parent's attitude was one of hypervigilant anxiety, the child, when grown, will behave in a similar fashion toward himself.

Treating the self as an object may also reflect early patterns of mother-child interaction for which there are no conscious memories. The effects of these interactions may persist in the psyche-soma. Christopher Bollas has called this the "unthought known."[44] Superimposed on the unthought known are memories of later interactions. Bollas provided several case histories that illustrate this principle. In one such example, he described a patient whose mother constantly fussed over her minor complaints and encouraged her to retreat from life instead of actively cope with it. Whenever this woman experienced the slightest touch of anxiety or depression in relation to work, a voice within her said, "Look, you don't have to take this kind of treatment—just tell them you don't feel well and go home."[45]

Self Representation and the "Objectification" of the Self

Structural theories of the self are designed to explain the fact that individuals have a continuing sense of identity. But in structural theory we encounter the philosophical problem of anthropomorphism. The concept of "self representation," introduced by Heinz Hartmann in 1950, was a return to a Cartesian "objectification" of the self.[46] Hartmann wished to avoid both Freud's anthropomorphism and the scientific problems inherent in a phenomenology of the self.

Although the term "self representation" did not figure in Freud's writings, Hartmann suggested that it was a natural extension of Freud's use of the term "object representation." Referring to the self as a self representation became fairly widespread in psychoanalytic thinking after 1950. The concept became an integral part of the theories of Jacobson and Kernberg, and it is still very much in current use within psychoanalysis.

Hartmann intended to correct Freud's failure to differentiate self from ego. He believed that the failure to differentiate self from ego contributed to a parallel confusion as to whether Freud intended the concept of narcissism to refer to the self or to the ego. "It therefore will be clarifying," he wrote, "if we define narcissism as the libidinal cathexis not of the ego but of the self. (It might also be useful to apply the term self-representation as opposed to object representation.)"[47]

Since Freud borrowed the concept of object representation from John Stuart Mill,[48] we must turn to philosophy to trace its origin. The philosopher Hilary Putnam has suggested that the meaning of a concept is not unlike a sense of personal identity, which, although modified through time, retains a certain continuity.[49] Thus, the concept "self and object representations," though altered within the context of psychoanalysis, retains some of its original meaning. Self and object representations are usually paired, in order to denote the presence or representation in the mind of a persistent and organized set of ideas and images regarding the self and other persons. When we speak of another's "self representation," we refer to the observer's construction of the subject's experience of self. Those who use these terms no doubt believe that they have "objectified" the self in a scientific manner.

The idea of a "presentation" within the mind derives from the Cartesian system of thought, in which objects in the external world have a perceptual representation within the self (mind). Implicit here is the idea that a self (another's consciousness) can be thought of as if it were an external object. The implication is that the self can be an object of perception by the self, as well as an object of perception by someone other than the self. In both instances, this object of perception can be called a "self representation." It is as if the mind's perception of the self were no different in kind from one's perception of a stone or of a cloud. Descartes observed that sensations produced by objects outside the self are presented to the mind.[50] He assumed that there was a similarity between objects external to the mind and their representation within the mind. Isaiah Berlin described the Cartesian notion of mind as follows: "The mind was something totally different in kind from the body which contained it like a box, in the part of itself called the brain." This led to a particular idea of mental representation: "Particles emanating from material objects strike the human sense organs, setting up a chain of effects in the nervous system, which somehow finally produces an entity different in kind from themselves—an idea in the mind."[51]

Freud attributed the idea of object representation to John Stuart Mill, who in turn borrowed the concept from John Locke. Locke did not question Descartes' assumption that there is a discrete, encapsulated, atomistic entity in the mind that represents the corresponding object in the real world. Taylor has described Locke's concept of self representation as "punctual," in the sense that it occupies a single point.[52] Locke believed that the mind is "wholly passive with respect to its simple ideas" and that there is a simple correspondence between physical objects and their representation in the mind.[53]

The term "self representation" denotes merely an inference that there are memories organized around ideas, affects, and images of the self. This concept does not solve the dilemma of the objectification of the self; it simply gives a name to the observer's inference of the subject's experience of self. One thus avoids the problem of anthropomorphism, but at the expense of creating a new difficulty. To suggest that a self representation is an entity in the individual's mind is an example of what James called the "psychologist's fallacy"—the confusion of the psychologist's own standpoint with that of the mental fact about which he is making his report.[54] James warned that the psychologist who reports on a presumed percept of the subject, such as a self representation, knows the self in *his* way and is easily misled into believing that this is the subject's experience.

Although a "representation" as described by Locke and later elaborated by Mill is atomistic and static, a passive point in the mind, it can be argued that the concept was effectively transformed when used in the context of psychoanalytic theory. One strikingly novel interpretation of self and object representations occurs in an influential paper by Joseph Sandler and Bernard Rosenblatt, "The Representational World."[55] They propose that self and object representations are the functional products of the ego. Furthermore, they view such representations not as fixed structures in the mind but as fluid creations of the child, as if the mind were a theater and the child were creating roles for the actors. In their hands the concept of self and object representations is not passive or atomistic. But it seems to me that they view self and object representations as descriptive of transitory, ephemeral experiences—as closer to states of consciousness than to psychic structures.

The term "self and object representations" has recently undergone still another change of meaning, in the field of infant research. Beatrice Beebe and Frank Lachmann use the concept to refer not to the conscious idea of an object but to an *unconscious* mental structure.[56] (For further discussion of this point see Chapter 6.) Beebe and Lachmann studied normal mother-infant interactions in babies aged three to four months. Using frame-by-frame analysis of film, they were able to observe rapid movements and affective expressions not easily visible to the eye. Most characteristically, the responses of mother and child were closely matched, suggesting a bond of unconscious communication. But even when the responses appeared to diverge, the disengagement was likewise coordinated. These coordinated responses were so rapid and subtle that one must assume they occurred unconsciously. Beebe and Lachmann suggested that as mother and child match each other's temporal and affective patterns, each recreates an inner psychophysiological state similar to that of the partner. They further suggested that positive matchings of this sort contribute to the "positive coloration of the self." It is not unreasonable to suppose that the confirmatory responses that validate the infant's affective states are internalized in healthy development and will contribute to the child's capacity to bring affective experiences within the domain of the self—within the domain of the personal. This synchrony of the affective states of mother and infant is bound to enhance the sense of continuity of the self in the infant, who is constantly experiencing rapid changes in mood and affect states.

William James: The Self as Pure Experience

According to James, experience is the fundamental datum that requires no further transposition into the domain of objectivity. He rejected Descartes' separation of the mind from the world, presenting an alternative to the Cartesian system which avoided the ego/self dilemma. In his essay "Does 'Consciousness' Exist?" he asks his reader to imagine the room in which he or she is reading.[57] He then argues that the ancient belief according to which a representation of the room exists in our mind, separate from the room itself, violates the reader's sense of life. Instead, he describes the perception of the room and the room itself as the intersection of different contexts, analogous to describing a point as the intersection between two lines. He further adds that each of these contexts, that of consciousness and that of the room itself, has a *historical* dimension (that is, a dimension within time): that of the reader's personal biography and that of the history of the house of which the room is a part. James summarizes his position as follows: "I think I may now claim to have made my thesis clear. Consciousness connotes a kind of external relation, and does not denote a special stuff or way of being. *The peculiarity of our experiences, that they not only are, but are known, which their 'conscious' quality is invoked to explain, is better explained by their relations—these relations themselves being experiences—to one another.*"[58]

James thus denied that consciousness denoted an *entity;* rather, he insisted that it stood for a *function. Consciousness is primarily a selecting agency, directing attention to what is most interesting.*[59] James also believed that consciousness had a "peculiar reference to a centre which we call the *self.*" I do not know whether one can improve upon James's description of the self and consciousness.

Consciousness includes a great deal more than consciousness of the self. For example, learning to drive a car initially requires one's conscious attention and interest, but only in a very peripheral sense does it require a consciousness of self. Such skills rapidly become an unconscious motor activity. We know that for some individuals, however, such motor acts do have great personal significance and meaning. Therefore, it is very difficult to distinguish consciousness from consciousness of self. In order to make this distinction possible, we must introduce the concepts of agency, value, and personal meaning, which will be discussed in Chapters 7 and 8. To paraphrase James's account of consciousness: *the self is a selecting agency, directing attention to that which has personal meaning.*

Like Freud's theory of the Oedipus complex and Fairbairn's theory of internal exciting and persecuting objects, James's notions of the self and of consciousness were inspired by his own intensely traumatic experiences. James, as is well known, suffered from a major depression which reached a point of crisis when he was twenty-eight years old, in 1870, one year after he graduated from Harvard Medical School. He had long known that he would not practice medicine, but he had not yet chosen his life's work. Following is his account of his aimless condition—a terrifying experience that proved to be pivotal in his life. The account is autobiographical, although it appears in *The Varieties of Religious Experience* disguised as a "translation from the French":

> Whilst in this state of philosophic pessimism and general depression of spirits about my prospects, I went one evening into a dressing-room in the twilight to procure some article that was there; when suddenly there fell upon me without any warning, just as if it came out of the darkness, a horrible fear of my own existence. Simultaneously there arose in my mind the image of an epileptic patient whom I had seen in the asylum, a black-haired youth with greenish skin, entirely idiotic, who used to sit all day on one of the benches, or rather shelves against the wall, with his knees drawn up against his chin, and the coarse grey undershirt, which was his only garment, drawn over them inclosing his entire figure. He sat there like a sort of sculptured Egyptian cat or Peruvian mummy, moving nothing but his black eyes and looking absolutely non-human. This image and my fear entered into a species of combination with each other. *That shape am I,* I felt potentially. Nothing that I possess can defend me against that fate, if the hour for it should strike me as it struck for him. There was such a horror of him, and such a perception of my own merely momentary discrepancy from him, that it was as if something hitherto solid within my breast gave way entirely, and I became a mass of quivering fear. After this the universe was changed for me altogether.[60]

Today, we can identify James's experience as a form of annihilation anxiety—a fear of losing the continuity and coherence of the self. James feared that his self could become disintegrated and that he was capable of being transformed into the idiotic epileptic that he viewed with such horror. The fear that one will lose the continuity of being and become transformed into someone else is the most severe form of anxiety that can afflict human beings. If an individual once experiences it, he or she will do anything, even commit suicide, to prevent a recurrence.[61]

I suggest that James's abiding interest in the phenomenology of the self, his life-long scanning of his consciousness, represents his attempt to avert annihilation anxiety by constant internal monitoring. After this episode, James gradually regained his health and found his life's work in psychology and philosophy. As Ralph Barton Perry remarked in his monumental work on William James, "His philosophy was never a mere theory, but always a set of beliefs that reconciled him to life . . . James required a philosophy to save him."[62]

It should be remembered that the Jamesian definition of consciousness does not coincide with Freud's idea that consciousness and the unconscious represent separate systems in the mind. James was interested in the dynamic unconscious and was fully aware that consciousness could be split, as in cases of multiple personalities. But he preferred Pierre Janet's explanation that the other self in multiple personalities represents a "second" consciousness. He did not believe in the existence of Freud's impersonal unconscious. James saw no point in calling something mental if it is not felt or experienced at least to some degree.[63] In this rejection of the unconscious as "nonmental," James was in accord with most of his colleagues. Freud may have been thinking of James when he said, "To most people who have been educated in philosophy the idea of anything psychical which is not also conscious is so inconceivable that it seems to them absurd and refutable simply by logic."[64]

James's description of the self was no less than panoramic.[65] He considered the self from three distinct aspects: first, the material, bodily self, which he called the *empirical* self; second, the social self; and third, the spiritual self, which he described as the core of the self, a "palpitating inward life, a central nucleus."[66] This core I would refer to as the *private* self; but James eschewed this term, for he wished to avoid the idea of a self entirely cut off from others. He retained a nearly mystical belief in the capacity of the self to communicate with other selves. In his later years he became absorbed in the problem of extrasensory perception and mental telepathy. Furthermore, he avoided the idea of a private self because he wished to separate empirical psychology from religious belief in a private soul that communicates only with God.

The social self is formed by the recognition of others. As James said, "Properly speaking, a man has as many social selves as there are individuals who recognize him and carry an image of him in their mind. To wound any one of these images is to wound him."[67] James's description has a very contemporary ring: your sense of self is contingent upon the *image* the other person has of you. (Compare Lacan's theory that the child identifies with the imaginary object of the mother's desire—the phallus.)

With regard to the core of the self, or the innermost, "spiritual" self, James recognized its multiple functions. This innermost self is the fountainhead of a personal morality, will power (motivation), and a creative apperception of the world. James described how, in the face of social opprobrium, the individual has recourse to his or her innermost self. Although the individual may crave social acceptance, *his or her inner ideal social self is the final judge and provides the ultimate accep-tance.* "When for motives of honor and conscience I brave the condemnation of my own family, club, and 'set'; when as a protestant I turn catholic; as a catholic freethinker; ... I am always inwardly strengthened in my course and steeled against the loss of my actual social self by the thought of other and better *possible* social judges than those whose verdict goes against me now ... The emotion that beckons me on is indu-bitably the pursuit of an ideal social self."[68]

James noted a paradox: that despite our dependence on so-cial affirmation, there is a portion of the self that enables us to become autonomous and free of such social dependency. James's "spiritual self," which I call the "private self," is the source of our deepest motivations and the source of our ulti-mate values. Our sense of well-being depends on the congru-ence between our actual self and the ideals to which we aspire. James knew that self esteem could be described by the follow-ing formula: *self esteem* = *success* divided by *pretensions.*[69]

The very act of introspection means that the self is an ob-ject to itself. There is an "I" that is witness to the "Me" as well as the "Not-Me." This "I" exists over time and is equated with a sense of identity that is a witness to the ephemeral "Me." James was very much aware of the para-dox of the continuity of the self amid a discontinuous stream of consciousness—a problem that he wrestled with until the end of his life without finding an adequate solution.

James and the Identity/Consciousness Paradox

As we have seen, Freud and Fairbairn accounted for the continuity of the self by positing that experience is frozen within the identifications of psychic structures. They did not consider the self in real time, the self as consciousness. James, in contrast, grasped the paradox of identity in its entirety. In *The Principles of Psychology,* James deals with the problem of reconciling a series of former selves with the self of current experience by proposing the following analogy.[70] He asks the reader to imagine a herd of cattle whose owner recognizes their "brand" as his own. These cattle (thoughts) may go their own way; the herd's unity is only a potential one until the owner arrives. The owner actively provides the coherence that underlies the sense of identity. But how does the owner impose this unity and coherence upon the herd? If consciousness is ever changing, how does one establish a unity between past and present? James suggests that "title" to the herd (thoughts) may be passed on from one owner to another, or to a succession of others (former selves). And "may not the 'title' of a collective self [an identity] be passed by one Thought to another in some analogous way?"[71] Here James links the experience of self to the question of time, to a historical dimension. He therefore emphasizes the centrality of time and the consciousness of self, as he did in his earlier paper "Does 'Consciousness' Exist?"

James later became dissatisfied with the "herdsman" analogy he presented in the *Principles* and continued to wrestle with the paradox of identity and consciousness. At the end of his life, he felt it to be nearly insoluble. Gerald Myers has related that James was unable to reconcile how a momentary state of consciousness could connect with the stored memories of previous selves and create the unity that we experience as identity. "James found many things mysterious—the nature of causality, the relation between mind and body, the concepts of continuity and infinity—but he encountered nothing more resistant to conceptualization than personal identity."[72]

I suspect that James would have welcomed Freud's theory of *Nachträglichkeit,* which posits that memory is a retranscription, that a retranslation of memory occurs as one enters successive developmental epochs. I discussed this subject in detail in *Other Times, Other Realities,*[73] where I pointed to the similarity between Freud's theory and Gerald Edelman's notion of memory as recategorization.[74] Edelman's theory of Neural Darwinism appears to have resolved the paradox that James believed insoluble.

Federn and the Phenomenology of the Self

Paul Federn, a member of the Psychological Wednesday Society and one of Freud's earliest supporters, was the first psychoanalyst to describe the conscious phenomenology of the self. He was a highly original thinker whose ideas about the self had little in common with Freud's concept of the ego. But Federn could not quite reconcile himself to his disagreements with Freud, since he was overawed by Freud and hesitated to challenge him openly. His attitude is expressed in marginal notes found in a book that he presented to a young colleague: "[You] shall be aware of my reluctance against changing or adding anything to Freud's presentations. I did it with deepest awe for his discoveries. Wherever I proceeded farther, I followed and did not leave behind his paths. I go with, not against, him—I had to do it because of my greater and better knowledge of the ego psychology."[75]

Federn's contribution has not received the attention it deserves because his unclear prose places a heavy burden on the reader. But, more important, in his effort to fit his observations into Freud's 1914 theory of narcissism, he obscured his own originality. His descriptions of the self were overlaid by Freud's theory of narcissism, expressed as the vicissitudes of libidinal cathexis.

Federn investigated the self phenomenologically, as did William James, but in keeping with Freud's terminology he referred to the "ego" rather than the "self."[76] Federn used the method of introspection to examine his experience of self in transitional states such as waking and falling asleep. In addition, he drew upon his knowledge gained as a pioneering psychotherapist of the psychoses. Like James, he observed that in healthy individuals the bodily self and the psychological self are unified. He suggested that the separation between the mental and bodily selves that is experienced in pathological states such as depersonalization contributed, developmentally, to the belief in the existence of a soul. He observed that in dreams the bodily self usually remains dormant, while various sectors of the mental self are fully represented.

Federn also believed that awareness of the continuity of the self is a primary psychological "given" that requires no further procedures such as the testing of reality.[77] As we shall see in Chapter 8, this assertion is supported by contemporary neurobiology; for the coherence and continuity of the self can be thought of as a homeostatic function, an evolutionary given. Federn spoke of this primal ego (self) feeling as follows: "an enduring feeling and knowledge that our ego is continuous and persistent, despite interruptions by sleep or unconsciousness, because we feel that processes within us, even though they may be interrupted by forgetting or unconsciousness, have a persistent origin within us, and that our body and psyche belong permanently to our ego."[78] Parallel to this enduring feeling of the self, Federn noted the normal existence of transient discontinuous "ego states." He believed that contradictory affective states can coexist in healthy individuals and do not threaten the sense of unity of the self. In addition to these transient ego states, the mind contains a record of archaic, primitive ego states that are normally repressed. In schizophrenia, where repression is undone, such primitive ego states become manifest.

Federn was responsible for introducing the concept of "ego boundaries." He viewed the differentiation of self from nonself as a very fluid process, because the self customarily enters into the object that it perceives. Federn noted a wide range of individual differences in the experience of ego boundaries, as well as daily fluctuations in boundary experiences within the same individual. Edith Jacobson believed that Federn exaggerated the extent to which normal persons project the self into the world.[79] But Jacobson's criticism may reflect the very point that Federn made— namely, that there are marked individual differences in the experience of ego boundaries. Indeed, there are some psychoanalysts who continue to believe that the experience of merging with another is a grave symptom of psychopathology, and not, as I maintain, an essential part of the dialectic of self and Other (see Chapter 4).

Didier Anzieu, a French psychoanalyst, recently reintroduced Federn's concept of fluid ego boundaries.[80] Anzieu invented the term "skin ego," a metaphor based on the bodily organ that differentiates self from nonself. Anzieu postulated that the infant's stroking of its own skin is probably the earliest opportunity the infant has to experience itself as an object. Touching the skin is experienced simultaneously as an internal and external sensation. Not only is the skin a boundary between self and nonself, but it also gives rise to this double representation.

Summary

I have used two central paradoxes as a means of organizing this overview of various theories of the self. One such paradox is that the self provides a continuity of being, yet is coterminus with an ever-changing consciousness. The self has therefore been viewed both as a psychic structure and as the center of consciousness. The second paradox is epistemological—one of the great paradoxes of modern philosophy, a seemingly insoluble puzzle. It is the problem of objectifying the subjective experience of self. Freud, I suggest, recognized this philosophical dilemma, but may not have fully grasped the implications of his own revolutionary solution. In his accounts of psychic structure, Freud shifted between a personal self in which structures were anthropomorphized and an impersonal ego in which psychic structures resulted from the neutralization of instinctual energy.

Freud did not consider the self as a center of consciousness; he described only the structural attributes of self. Most psychoanalysts, with the exception of Federn and Kohut, have followed Freud in investigating only the structural wing of this paradox. When describing psychic structures as persons, Freud depicted two somewhat different conditions. In the first instance, an identification with the other person replaces the self; in the second, the entire *relationship* between the self and the object in the external world is transposed into the self.

Freud's observation that a *relationship* between the self and the object can be transposed from the external world into the self became the starting point of Fairbairn's theory of endopsychic structures. Like Freud, Fairbairn viewed the structures of the self as internalizations of relationships. But in Fairbairn's theory, structures are records of traumatic interactions, whereas for Freud, psychic structures represented a mosaic of lost objects. Fairbairn considered the self only in its structural context, ignoring the attributes of the self as consciousness, the self in real time. In contrast to Freud, he did not shift from an impersonal ego to a personal self but instead dealt with the self/ego dilemma by a totally explicit anthropomorphism of internalized object relations.

It can be stated as a general principle that traumatic relationships in the external world are transposed and recreated within the self, so that the self always contains within it subject and object.

The concept of "self representation" was introduced by Hartmann, who evidently believed that Freud's failure to differentiate self from ego was resolvable if one could describe an objectified self. By using the concept of self representation, Hartmann hoped to avoid Freud's anthropomorphism. A self representation considered in this fashion would then be no different in kind from any other object of perception: it is an outside observer's inference of the subject's self experience. In this light, it seems to me that Freud's double characterization of self and ego is a more subtle method of coping with the self/ego dilemma. I believe that Freud's anthropomorphic characterizations of the structures of the self were absolutely necessary in order to depict the personal relationships that contribute to the inner self. The subject's experience of self is not an object of perception that is on the same footing as other objects in the external world. Thus, I consider the concept of self representation, when it refers to the idea of an object, to be retrogressive.

William James is perhaps the only major theorist who fully grasped both wings of the paradox: the self as a mental structure and the self as consciousness. James believed that the self is the center of consciousness, yet he was fully aware of the structural aspect of self as an identity persisting through time. Despite all his efforts, the solution to the paradox eluded him.

According to James, Descartes' belief that a representation of an object exists in our mind, distinct from the object itself, violates a sense of life. Rather, experience is the fundamental datum that requires no further transposition into the domain of objectivity. James's phenomenology of the self implies certain divisions or polarities of the self, which I shall elaborate in the next chapter: first, the self is grounded in biology—the self is a bodily self; second, there is an innermost self that is the origin of self sufficiency, of a sustaining personal morality, and of our deepest motivations; third, there is a social self that is formed by the recognition of others.

2

Private and Public Selves

> Each individual is an isolate, permanently non-communicating, permanently unknown, in fact unfound.
>   DONALD W. WINNICOTT, *Maturational Processes and the Facilitating Environment*

My concept of the private self is rooted in biology and is congruent with Gerald Edelman's theory of the self as a value-laden memory system. Here I would like to show that the tendency to minimize the importance of the private self can be traced to a conviction held by some authors that the self is essentially disembodied. This is true, for example, of the philosopher George Herbert Mead, whose view of the self has influenced generations of sociologists and social scientists. It is also true of Heinz Kohut and the school of self psychology that he founded.

This chapter presents observations from psychoanalysis, infant research, and neurobiology that illustrate the vital significance of the private self. In contemporary psychoanalysis, Winnicott was the first to recognize fully the importance of the private self. Yet Winnicott also emphasized that the private self owes its existence to the facilitating maternal environment, a dependency that generates the following paradox: *to become autonomous, one needs the presence of another.* We possess both autonomous private selves and dependent social selves, which appear to have opposing aims. In psychoanalysis in recent years, perhaps due to the growing interest in object relatedness, the self-generating aspect of the self has been deemphasized in favor of the view that the individual owes his or her coherence of self to another person, which Kohut calls the "selfobject." But neurobiology and infant research suggest a very different conclusion.

Whether one believes that a private self is essentially self created or, conversely, that the self is primarily bestowed upon the individual by others reflects one's attitudes toward the individual and society. If one believes that seeking validation from others is a fundamental human aspiration, then one depicts a self that has the potential to be in harmony with society and free of intergenerational strife and conflict. This is an explicit theme in Kohut's self psychology. Kohut criticized Freud for choosing Oedipus, a parricide, as the central mythic figure of psychoanalysis. He would have chosen Odysseus, who, according to myth, saved his son's life.[1] Kohut viewed self psychology as essentially conflict free and contrasted his views of the self with those of researchers such as René Spitz and Margaret Mahler, who believed in a "nuclear self," a self motivated toward individuation. As Kohut wrote, "I can perhaps point up the difference of outlook most sharply by stating that from the point of view of the psychoanalytic psychology of the self, a value-laden demand for psychological independence is nonsense—almost as nonsensical as would be a demand that the human body should be able to get along without oxygen."[2]

From one perspective, the self is self generating: it bootstraps itself into existence. But this bootstrapping requires the presence and empathic synchrony of another. The paradox is that in order to become relatively autonomous, one requires—in childhood and for the rest of one's life—some degree of affirmation from another. But self affirmation and self actualization are not achieved without conflict, in contrast to what Kohut would claim; they are achieved by struggling *against* the other. My own conviction is that if indeed there is a hierarchy of human aspirations, self actualization through the emergence of personal values and personal interests takes precedence over social affirmation. I thus emphasize the centrality of the private self. This is, of course, a view from the West; Eastern societies such as India, China, and Japan, which deemphasize self actualization, have found other means of achieving continuity and coherence of the self. But if one believes that the self is created primarily by society (Mead) or bestowed through the mirroring of the child's caretakers (Kohut), one will consider the existence of a private self to be of secondary importance.

There is some support from contemporary neuroscience for the view that the autonomy of the self is fundamental.[3] Edelman has ascribed to the self the function of allowing the individual to become relatively autonomous from the tyranny of events in real time. The primacy of the quest for self actualization is also supported by the work of Kurt Goldstein, a neuropathologist who studied brain-damaged individuals from a holistic point of view. Goldstein thought deeply about human nature and came to the conclusion that there was only one drive, that of self actualization:

> Since the tendency to actualize itself as fully as possible is the basic drive, the only drive by which the sick organism is moved, and since the life of the normal organism is determined in the same way, it is clear that the goal of the drive is not a discharge of tension, and that we have to assume only one drive, the drive of self-actualization. Under various conditions various actions come into the foreground; and since they seem thereby to be directed to-

wards different goals, they give the impression of existing independently of each other. [These actions occur] in accordance with the various capacities which belong to the nature of the organism, and in accordance with those instrumental processes which are the necessary prerequisites for the self-actualization of the organism.[4]

The Embodied Self

James referred to the bodily self as the "empiric" self. The fact that the self is embodied is supported by the commonplace observation that what we may find disgusting in others we easily accept in ourselves; this is especially true with regard to our feces and bodily odors. Freud likewise asserted that "the ego is first and foremost a bodily ego: it is not merely a surface entity, but is itself the projection of a surface."[5] Paul Schilder, in *The Image and Appearance of the Human Body,* investigated the self as a projected schema of the body; the body image is one of the organizers of the experience of self.[6] The effect of the absence of such a visual image of the body has been noted by John Hull, who became totally blind in adulthood and experienced a loss in the continuity of self, because he lacked the ability to see the outlines of his body: "One can't glance down and see the reassuring continuity of one's own consciousness in the outlines of one's own body, moving a distant foot which, so to speak, waves back, saying, 'Yes, I hear you, I am here.'"[7]

Phyllis Greenacre believed that the body areas which contribute most to a sense of identity and which are particularly subject to distortion are the face and the genitals, and to a lesser extent the total bodily configuration.[8] Greenacre, like Schilder, viewed the body image as the core of the self, an image that is relatively stable but subject to the influence of mood. This body schema is reorganized at nodal points in childhood development and also in the adult life cycle. We know that when individuals believe they have a defective self, they are most likely to experience this as a defect in the body, and vice versa. When individuals think of themselves as defective, their perception of their body can sometimes assume a quasi-delusional character (from the perspective of an outside observer).

Edelman's Neurobiological Self

To the best of my knowledge, Gerald Edelman was the first to advance a model of the self as an evolutionary structure. In his book *Neural Darwinism,* Edelman proposes a theory of memory that fits in very well with psychoanalytic observations.[9] It is not necessary, he says, to posit a record in the central nervous system that is isomorphic with past experience. Instead, he suggests that memory consists of a recategorization of experience. This concept is similar to Freud's idea of *Nachträglichkeit,* a theory of memory that Freud introduced quite early in the history of psychoanalysis. Freud, like Edelman, considered memory to be a retranscription. In *The Remembered Present,* Edelman presents a model of the biological self.[10] Taking a Jamesian perspective, he views the self as nearly coterminous with consciousness: consciousness implies the capacity for self/nonself discrimination.[11] The evolution of higher-order consciousness (in humans and in other advanced species) confers on the individual a distinct adaptive advantage because it *enables the organism to be free from the tyranny of ongoing events in real time.* "In higher-order consciousness, the emergence of concepts and, later, of symbolism allows the use of memory to develop *a coherent picture or an internal model of present, past and future.* It seems likely that complex demands for recognition and action—whether to leap from one branch to another or to recognize a predator—provided a strong selective force for the evolutionary development of various neural systems that free an animal from the dominance of an immediate driven response."[12]

If the self contributes to the individual's inclusive fitness by freeing the individual from the tyranny of real time, it follows that separate neural structures must have evolved which generate the experience of self in contrast to the experience of the world. The experience of self is linked to the salience of perception, which in turn derives from evolutionary givens described as "value." According to Edelman, "value-dependent behaviors require the operation of specific portions of the nervous system that differ structurally and functionally from those carrying out perceptual categorizations."[13] The self exists, according to Edelman, to assure the dominance of adaptive homeostasis. It has not been sufficiently recognized that these two parts of the central nervous system differ radically in their evolution. Edelman believes, therefore, that a self/nonself discrimination is structurally inherent in the central nervous system of those species who possess higher-order consciousness. "The functioning of such a system," Edelman states, "can determine the relative salience of external events according to *internal value schemes.*"[14] The self system is oriented internally and based on introspection; it exerts a selective bias that determines what, in consciousness, *is of interest to the individual.* Edelman identifies these structures as follows: "Self is fundamentally determined by the signalling activity of areas mediating homeostatic—autonomic, hedonic, neuroendocrine—brain functions. Such areas include brain stem and pontine nuclei, mesencephalic reticular formation, hypothalamus, amygdala, septum and fornix, and their various connections to prelimbic forebrain areas. In contrast, nonself signals are composed of corticothalamic inputs and of cerebellar and hippocampal loops other than those in the fornical path."[15]

I consider higher-order consciousness and the self to be nearly equivalent. But, as I have indicated, consciousness includes more than consciousness of self. Edelman's model of higher-order consciousness, which provides a coherent model of past, present, and future, is largely congruent with psychoanalytic observation: the continuity and coherence of the self is a homeostatic requirement of the psyche-soma. The psychoanalyst is best positioned to observe the pathology of the self, defined as all that impedes the development of this coherence. This is seen in the phenomena described as the "splitting" of the self and the "decentering" of the self. Of special importance for the psychoanalysis of the self is the concept of "value."

The self is the repository of a value-laden memory system. As Edelman has written: "Current perceptual events are recategorized in terms of past value-category matches. It is the *contrast* of the special linkage of value and past categories with currently arriving categories, and the *dominance* of the self-related special memory systems in this memorial linkage, that generate the self-referential aspect of consciousness."[16] This value-laden memory system, persisting over time, interacts with the environment, through reentrant signaling, in real time.[17] As Edelman notes, *this self-related memory system generates a self-referential aspect of consciousness.* Edelman thus offers a model which promises to resolve the paradox that William James thought insoluble: continuity of the self as identity and discontinuity of the self in the flux of consciousness. The continuity of the self is preserved by means of the self's linkage with the homeostatic brain systems. The paradox is resolved through reentry and recategorization. Perceptions occurring in real time are recategorized through a "matching" with the value-laden memories of former states. A sense of the continuity of the self amid the flux of perception is assured, because the self acts as a dominant template imposing order and coherence on current perception.

Edelman's model therefore encompasses the interaction between the relatively stable memories of the self and the ephemeral experience of consciousness in real time. He posits the existence of value-laden memorial systems that are in constant interaction with the perception of the world. Edelman stresses the importance of action in perception: "Because perceptual categorizations are driven by action, and because they are in constant interaction with systems carrying out conceptual categorizations, the continuity of consciousness is assured. Reentry, which has a strong temporal and rhythmic character, also contributes to both continuity and change, yielding Jamesian properties."[18]

Edelman's biological theory of the self is based on a biology of individual differences. Although consciousness of the self requires specific neural structures that are shared within a given species, memories are the record of the experience of an *individual*. There are enormous variations within the central nervous system, with regard to both structure and function, that cannot be attributed to genetic information. The brain can be thought of as an organ unlike any other, in that it is tailor-made for the individual. The self generates emergent and highly individualized values, which undoubtedly reflect this tailor-made structure.

Edelman indicates that the nervous system is not as genetically hard-wired as had been previously supposed— that even within the constraints of genetic instruction, the embryological development of the nervous system shows a remarkable degree of variability from the level of the cell to the level of global functioning. This variability results from a dynamic interaction with the environment. Not only do significant variations in morphology arise in this manner, but the functional organization of the central nervous system is also dynamically responsive to the environment at every level of organization. This means that genetically identical twins, even at birth, do not perceive the world identically. Each person perceives the world in a unique way—that is to say, every individual constructs his or her own reality. Modern science has confirmed what William Blake apprehended intuitively: "A fool sees not the same tree that a wise man sees."

Oliver Sacks, in a review of Edelman's theory of Neural Darwinism, made a similar observation: "Darwin provided a picture of the evolution of species; Edelman has provided a picture of the evolution of the individual nervous system, as it reflects the life experience of each individual human being. The nervous system adapts, is tailored, evolves so that experience, will, sensibility, moral sense, and all that one would call personality or soul becomes engraved in the nervous system. The result is that one's brain is one's own. One is not an immaterial soul, floating around in a machine. I do not feel alive, psychologically alive, except insofar as a stream of feeling—perceiving, imagining, remembering, reflecting, revising, recategorizing—runs through me. I am that stream—that stream is me."[19]

The attributes of the biological self can be summarized as follows: The biological self is the repository of value-laden long-term memories that provide a measure of autonomy from perceptual inputs in real time. By means of concepts and symbolic representations (a higher-order level of consciousness), individuals have access to a coherent internal model of past, present, and future. This coherence is an inestimable aid in learning complex tasks, but it must also be considered a homeostat.

The implications of Edelman's biological self are manifold. Marked individual differences in the development of the central nervous system support a "constructivist's" view of multiple realities. In a certain sense, we create our worlds through a kind of internal bootstrapping. It is a model that resolves the paradox of the self as both identity and consciousness. The biological self is the foundation of individuality; it is both self creating and self actualizing. Biology can now be seen as the source of personhood.

The Self and Mastery

Edelman's demonstration that self/nonself differentiation is mediated by specific neural structures implies that this differentiation is present in infancy. The infant's capacity to differentiate self from nonself can, in fact, be confirmed by direct observation, as summarized by Daniel Stern.[20] For example, he observed Siamese twins who sucked each other's fingers yet were able to differentiate their own hands from those of the other. Stern describes an early core of the self, in which the infant is aware that it is the agent of action. A sense of the continuity of being is established through action, which is experienced as joyful. Edelman's theory of Neural Darwinism suggests that individuals, through action, seek to reestablish categorical memories. Stern suggests something similar and refers to invariable interpersonal interactions, which he calls "representations of interactions that have been generalized" (RIGs). The experience of self is inseparable from *activity*.

As all observers of children and animals have noted, there is joy in those activities that result in an experience of mastery. Robert White calls this experience one of *efficacy*

and *competence*.[21] It is important to recognize that this pleasure is different from the pleasures of relatedness or the
pleasure of consummatory activities such as eating a good
meal or having sex.[22] T. Berry Brazelton calls this "fueling
the system from within."[23] I believe that this capacity to find
joy from within, through mastery, remains a core of the private self. When it is present, the self feels strong; when it is
absent, the self feels weak and depleted.

In his essay "Ego and Reality in Psychoanalytic Theory,"
White develops the idea that activities can be satisfying in
themselves and not for specific consequences: "My thesis is
that the seeking of efficacy is a primitive biological endowment as basic as the satisfactions that accompany feeding or
sexual gratification."[24] I would add that such joys can be experienced in solitude, when the other is absent or is merely a
silent presence (see Chapter 5).

Researchers have noted that infants are able to regulate
their interactions with their mothers, so that periods of relatedness alternate with periods of nonrelatedness. Louis
Sander refers to this private time as "open space."[25] Sander
and his collaborators observed newborn infants interacting
with their mothers in an around-the-clock longitudinal
study. They found that by the third week of a child's life, the
mother responds to the infant's needs by providing it with
periods of relative disengagement. Sander sees this as the infant's opportunity to exercise an "individually idiosyncratic
and selective volitional initiative." The infant is free to follow its own *interests,* which may involve self-exploration
or responses to low-level stimuli. Sander makes the very
significant point that *disengagement and engagement hold
places of equal importance.*

Researchers largely agree that the infant needs to maintain active control over which aspects of the core self will be
shared with others.[26] There is thus widespread recognition

that a private self exists within the infant.[27] This is not to imply, however, that the infant's private self can exist without a facilitating maternal environment. Some researchers refer to the private self as the "I", which is to be distinguished from the social self, the "We."[28] One might infer that in contemporary psychoanalytic theory the importance of the infant's private space has been overlooked in the emphasis on relatedness. In this context, the negativism of the two-year-old has been understood as an attempt to reestablish this private space. René Spitz viewed the infant's head-shaking, signaling "no," as the first indication of the infant's exercising independent judgment—what it wishes to take in or to expel.[29]

In adults, an absence of a sense of efficacy results in a sense of futility and a depressive lowering of self esteem. Fairbairn believed that this sense of futility is the characteristic affect of a self that is dissociated or split.[30] The sense of futility is often associated with an absence of meaning, an indication that the individual has become decentered from his or her private self (see Chapter 3). Winnicott likewise observed that when one is immersed in a false self, there is a sense of unreality and futility.[31] This inability to believe in one's efficacy can pervade the entire personality. People with such feelings are convinced that they can never make things happen.

Edward Bibring believed that the depressions of everyday life result from the ego's sense of helplessness. Depression, he claimed, represents a basic reaction to situations of narcissistic frustration which are beyond the power of the ego to master.[32]

If mastery is a source of joy and if the failure of mastery results in a sense of hopelessness and despair, there are powerful motives to extend the hegemony of the self. "Efficacy of the self" refers not only to action in the world but also to the inner capacity to maintain the integrity of the self in the face of painful incursions of affects and impulses. Intensity of feeling from whatever source may be threatening, but there is some gain in recognizing these feelings to be part of the self. If the self can experience such incursions as something within its own control, the self is strengthened. Winnicott referred to this process when he spoke of the way in which an id impulse can either disrupt a weak ego or strengthen a strong one.[33] If intense affective experiences can be contained within the self, the self extends its domain and the individual will feel strengthened, alive, and authentic.

Some puzzling fantasies and behaviors, which might be labeled perverse, can be understood as an attempt to extend this hegemony of the self over these intense and intrusive affects. For example, the self can extend its control by means of eroticization, experiencing sexuality in contexts that are not usually recognized as erotic. It is well known that hatred can become eroticized, so that some perversions can be understood as the erotic form of hatred.[34] It is also well known that anxiety can become eroticized, and that the fear of being totally controlled by another can become converted into erotic desire. To the extent that others can control the self through the threat of humiliation, the feeling of humiliation can likewise be eroticized. For example, one patient of mine feared that a "defect" within herself would be exposed to others and that she would then be subjected to overwhelming shame and humiliation. Her "defect" consisted of the fact that if she became intensely anxious, she might begin to shake and her anxiety would thereby be exposed for all to see. She lived in constant fear that this "defect" would be revealed. She reported that during masturbation she fantasized she was in diapers and had a bowel movement in her underpants in public. This fantasy undoubtedly had multiple determinants, but one meaning is evident: by eroticizing this humiliation in fantasy, she was able to bring the humiliation within the hegemony of the self.

Winnicott's "True" and "False" Selves

Winnicott was one of the few psychoanalysts who recognized the existence of both private (true) and social (false) selves. Winnicott emphasized the unity of the psyche-soma: the true self is a somato-psychic phenomenon, and not simply a psychological entity.[35] The true self is the locus of the infant's first creative action, which Winnicott called the "spontaneous gesture." The spontaneous gesture can be viewed as the precursor of the creation of private meanings. It is a gesture that arises from the baby alone. Though the mother may impede or facilitate the infant's spontaneous gestures, in this activity the child is not mirroring the mother but is creating something that is independent of the mother. The spontaneous gesture is, then, a paradigm for the child's independent and wholly individualistic apperception of the world. If the development of the true self is not impaired, the infant has an assured sense of being real, of being psychically alive. Winnicott believed that this capacity for creative apperception is essential for mental health: "It is creative apperception more than anything else that makes the individual feel that life is worth living."[36] Winnicott also observed: "We find either that individuals live creatively and feel that life is worth living or else they cannot live creatively and are doubtful about the value of living. The variable in human beings is directly related to the quality and quantity of environmental provision at the beginning."[37]

Impairment of the development of the true self can come from within or from without. Those mothers who do not allow for their infant's creativity, claimed Winnicott, are "doing something worse than castration."[38] Impairment of the true self can also come from within, if intense internal stimuli, such as those attributable to instincts, are not brought within the experience of the true self. Here again, this is a process that the mother can either facilitate or impede.[39] Winnicott suggested that if internal stimuli can be brought within the experience of the true self, the child can react without being traumatized. The infant experiences pleasure in mastering internal stimuli in the same way it experiences pleasure in learning to walk. The private self, therefore, is the locus not only of creativity but also of the joy of mastery.

Winnicott viewed the false or social self as a defensive structure that protects the authenticity of the true self by social compliance. Communications that have their source within the false self do not feel real. But a certain degree of social compliance is necessary: "In the healthy individual who has a compliant aspect of the self but who exists and who is a creative and spontaneous being, there is at the same time a capacity for the use of symbols. In other words health here is closely bound up with the capacity of the individual to live in an area that is intermediate between the dream and reality, that which is called cultural life."[40] Winnicott believed that a reliable ego support consists of a mother who supports the infant's spontaneity—supports the spontaneous gesture. If the true self is exploited by the other, it will be annihilated, and it must therefore defend itself against such exploitation at all costs. According to Winnicott, it is more accurate to say the false self hides the infant's inner reality than to say it hides the true self.[41] He saw the true self as a bodily self that preserves a sense of the continuity of being, the loss of which is psychic death.[42] "The central [true] self could be said to be the inherited potential which is experiencing a continuity of being, and acquiring in its own way a personal psychic reality and a personal body-scheme. It seems necessary to allow for the concept of the isolation of this central self as a characteristic of health. Any threat to this isolation of the true self constitutes a major anxiety at this early stage, and defenses of earliest infancy appear in relation to failures of maternal care to ward off impingements which might disturb this isolation."[43]

In summary, then, Winnicott described a polarity between the true and false selves. The true self, the bodily self, is the source of authenticity, psychic aliveness, and the assurance of the continuity of being. The false self responds compliantly to others in order to protect the true self from nonacceptance and exploitation. The true self is paradoxical in that it enables the individual to be alone but requires initially the continuity of the external environment—that is to say, the presence of the mother. In his account of the mother's mirror role, Winnicott viewed this attunement as "the mother's role of giving back to the baby the baby's own self."[44] Finally, the true self can be totally private and noncommunicating. "I am putting forward and stressing the importance of the idea of the *permanent isolation of the individual* and claiming that at the core of the individual there is no communication with the not-me world."[45]

I do not accept Winnicott's terminology of "true" self and "false" self, essentially for two reasons. First, I believe the aspect of privacy is more salient than that of authenticity; and, second, I believe the term "true" connotes something that is a homogenous entity. As Richard Rorty has remarked, Freud's view of the psyche is such that each part is an equally plausible candidate for the "true self."[46] Furthermore, Rorty attacks the very idea of a "true" self, since it suggests a generalized standard of how a person should be, as opposed to a particularized individual self. On the other hand, the term "private self" connotes not an essence but a particularized experience.

Kohut's "Selfobject"

Since the tenets of Kohut's self psychology are well known, I shall not attempt here any systematic or comprehensive review of his ideas. But my work is in part a response to the one-sidedness of his theory. Kohut's self is nearly exclusively a social self, a self dependent on a selfobject for survival. Kohut does not recognize the need for self actualization, apart from the selfobject. That is, he does not recognize the existence of a self-generating self that could, in Brazelton's words, "fuel itself" from within. Kohut's failure to recognize the generative capacity of the self has been noted by Paul Ricoeur, who asks us to imagine how a self with no external support could survive. Ricoeur's answer is: by defining itself as living, as enjoying itself, as identifying with itself by means of this enjoyment.[47] This is a recognition of a private self which is essentially self creating.

Although Kohut avoids proposing a definition of the self, he emphasizes that the self and the selfobject form a complete system. Kohut states, in effect, that there is no self without a selfobject. The self therefore can be implicitly defined by the selfobject, which supplies to the self its cohesion, firmness, and harmony.[48] Kohut's clearest definition of the selfobject appears in a letter to a colleague: "The maxim that the self requires a milieu of empathically responding selfobjects in order to function, *indeed in order to survive,* applies not only in the instances of selves who because of unusual talents and skills are able to express their pattern in a form that has broad social consequences (such as in the cases of O'Neill and Proust), it is even more valid in the case of anonymous Everyman." Kohut eschews the concepts of independence and individuation, which he believes belong to a very different world view with a different set of values: "I can perhaps point up the difference of outlook most sharply by stating that from the point of view of the psychoanalytic psychology of the self a value-laden demand for psychological independence is nonsense—almost as nonsensical as would be the demand that the human body should be able to get along without oxygen."[49]

A similar description of the selfobject has been provided by Kohut's collaborator, Ernest Wolf. In his view, the cohesion of the self is provided for by the *environment*. Even the autonomy of the self is seen as a secondary effect of the selfobject. There is no indication that the cohesion of the self may be self generated. "Proper selfobject experiences favor the structural *cohesion* and energic *vigor* of the self; *faulty* selfobject experiences facilitate the *fragmentation* and *emptiness* of the self. Along with food and oxygen, every human being requires age-appropriate selfobject experiences from infancy to the end of life. The self cannot exist as a cohesive structure—that is, cannot generate an experience of well being—apart from the contextual surround of appropriate selfobject experiences."[50]

Kohut recognizes certain polarities within the self, but these polarities do not correspond to the distinction between the private self and the social self.[51] He describes a "bipolar" self, consisting of a "grandiose-exhibitionistic" self and a self that finds wholeness through a merger with an idealized selfobject. When the individual is under the sway of the grandiose self, the selfobject is experienced as a mirror or a twin of the grandiose self. When the individual seeks wholeness through a merger with an idealized selfobject, the self may be experienced as small and diminished in comparison with the idealized selfobject. In the nondefective self, where there is psychic health, Kohut claims there is an "uninterrupted tension arc" from basic ambitions, via basic talents and skills, toward basic ideals. This is an acknowledgment of a generative process within the self, but this generative process is dependent upon the selfobject.[52]

Kohut has been extensively criticized for his failure to recognize that many antecedents of his observations can be found in the work of Rank, Fairbairn, Winnicott, Mahler, and others.[53] When I first encountered Kohut's self psychology, it seemed to me that he was rediscovering and presenting in dramatic form certain aspects of the psychology of the self that were familiar to psychoanalysts who worked with sicker patients, especially analysts identified with the British school of object relations. I therefore remained skeptical of his claim that self psychology represented a radically new psychology which could not be integrated into Freudian psychoanalysis. I have come to adopt a different point of view: *what is radical in self psychology is not its clinical observations but its philosophical position.* When confronted with the dilemma of the ego and the self, Kohut did not follow Freud, who dealt with the ego/self dilemma by shifting from one domain to the other. For Kohut, the primacy of empathic understanding, defined as a vicarious introspection, is an irreducible given. Kohut therefore shuns all attempts to "objectify" the experience as a self representation. His stance is not unlike that of William James, for whom the subjective experience of consciousness required no further objectification. Kohut's position is also not unlike that of Giambattista Vico, who believed that there is a sense in which we can know more about the experience of others, in which we participate, than we can ever know about nonhuman nature, which we can only observe from the outside.[54]

Kohut might be described as a radical phenomenologist.[55] As Marilyn Nissim-Sabat has noted, Kohut's conviction that empathy is a fundamental form of knowledge is similar to the position taken by Husserl.[56] Husserl believed that consciousness in itself "has a being of its own which is absolutely unique, that it becomes in fact the field of a new science, that of phenomenology."[57] Through acts of immediate intuition, we intuit a "self." Kohut makes a similar claim for self psychology: "As I have stated repeatedly since 1959 when I first clarified my operational position, I do not believe we are dealing with separate biological and psychological universes, but with two approaches to reality. When science approaches reality via extrospection (and vicarious extrospection), we call it physics or biology; when it approaches it via introspection (and empathy), we call it psychology."[58]

That Kohut's position can be justifiably described as a radical phenomenology is illustrated by his comments regarding the topic of object loss. For Freud, the loss of the object is the motive for structure formation; most psychoanalysts believe that object loss is central to any human psychology. John Bowlby, in his monumental studies of attachment and loss, demonstrated that, as children, we share with our fellow primates an evolutionary heritage resulting in a common reaction to loss and separation.[59] Yet the topic of object loss does not appear in Kohut's self psychology.[60] The topic of object loss, in Kohut's view, belongs to biology, to the world of "extrospection" and hence has no place in self psychology: "I have said many times since in various ways ... that the archaic selfobject need did not proceed from the loss of a love object but from the loss of a more mature selfobject experience."[61] I interpret Kohut's statement to mean that from the standpoint of self psychology the only relevant data are the subjective experiences of the self. The loss of the object "in reality" is a subject for biology and not psychology. I believe that this radical position illustrates the limitations of phenomenology in general and of self psychology in particular. In a sense, Kohut's phenomenology of the self is the antithesis of Hartmann's notion of self representation; neither provides a solution to the self/ego dilemma, and both are clinically and philosophically indefensible.

Other Perspectives on the Private and Social Selves

The idea of a private self may be very ancient, for Aristotle recognized that we can achieve autonomy through a passionate commitment to personal moral values. Aristotle observed that although we are not masters of our impulses, we are in control of our moral choices—our *prohairesis.* "The tyrant says: I will put you in bonds. 'What are you saying? Put *me* in bonds? You will fetter my leg, but not even Zeus can conquer my *prohairesis.*'"[62] One's soul cannot be enslaved.

Although the term "soul" and the Greek term "psyche" are interchangeable, the Platonic and early Christian idea of a soul refers to that part of the psyche that is private and communicates only with God. It seems to me that the idea of a soul, in this sense, is not too different from the idea of a private self. Alasdair MacIntyre, however, makes a distinction between the Platonic idea of a soul and the idea of a soul that is associated with Catholic Christianity. In the former case the soul has an identity that precedes bodily and social existence, whereas in Catholic Christianity the soul has a role in a heavenly *community* represented on earth by the Church.[63]

Our modern view is that one can remain free so long as one is in contact with this inner, private self, which is self sustaining. This inner self, whether viewed as a private self or as a soul, is an alternate means of being in the world. As Aristotle observed, the freedom to make moral choices raises one above an unpropitious environment.[64]

The modern idea of a "true," inner self which is the fount not only of moral values but of authenticity is an idea we owe to Saint Augustine.[65] He introduced the idea of a private self capable of self reflection and furthermore, believed that acceptance and understanding of this private self intimate a love of the self.[66] In this, Augustine envisioned the very contemporary idea that self knowledge leads to self acceptance, a healthy form of self love that is obscured by the overburdened term "narcissism."

There is, however, a countervailing contemporary view of the self—namely, that the self owes its very existence to the other or to the collective social "others." The philosopher George Herbert Mead believed that one first experiences oneself as an object of others: "The organism does not become an entity to itself except in a social context; it does not get into the environment except through the social process. There is no self unless there is the possibility of regarding it as an object to itself."[67] According to this view, the self is formed by an assimilation of the (collective) attitudes of other individuals toward that self. Selfhood, according to Mead, is not created; it is bestowed upon the individual from without.[68]

The Self of George Herbert Mead

The views of George Herbert Mead have had considerable influence among social scientists and interpersonal psychiatrists, including Harry Stack Sullivan. Mead's self is not an individualized self but a self formed by society; like the self of William James, Freud, and Fairbairn, it contains both subject and object. But Mead believed that the self discovers itself only as an object: the self first appears through the mediation of another.[69] It is a self that reproduces external relationships within itself. The similarity to psychoanalytic theories of the self may end at this point, however. For Mead's description is an account of the process of socialization that the child experiences in relation to its peers in games and play. He thus depicts a much later developmental stage, when compared to the emergence of self in infancy that I have described. Although Mead acknowledges the bodily self, he does not see the coherence of the self as a biologically determined homeostatic requirement; instead, the unity of the self is bestowed upon the individual by society. "The organism as a whole becomes part of the environment only as it is involved in the social process. The organism does not become an entity to itself except in a social context. The self involves a unity; it is there in the social process, but there is no self unless there is the possibility of regarding it as an object to itself."[70]

According to Mead, the self is formed through experimental play in which one imitates or mirrors the roles of others. From the many roles assumed, there gradually arises a "generalized" other. This generalized other is a kind of corporate individual, a composite photograph which the self composes of other members of its society.[71] The self arises through social communication, through language; one takes on the role of the generalized other and acts toward oneself as others do.

Mead sees this generalized other, this "Me," as the core of the self. What corresponds to the private self is Mead's "I," a spontaneously arising critical faculty that challenges the values of the socialized "Me." Mead's nuclear self is the opposite of my conception of the private self, in that it is not self created and noncommunicating but is a collection of roles which the individual is assigned by society. The biologically given uniqueness of the individual is "transcended"; wholeness is something bestowed from the outside, and in turn this generalized other exercises control over individuality. Individuality is thus submerged in this generalized other. Mead, however, recognizes that the individual is not totally submissive to the generalized other. There is another polarity within the self: the "I," which is rooted in the individual's biological equipment. The "I" includes the relatively free, unpredictable, and creative portion of the self. But because Mead places the "Me" at the center of the self and the "I" on the periphery as a critical observer, his "collective" self is not an individual. So that despite Mead's acknowledgment of the influence of biology upon the self, his theory of the self is essentially disembodied.

Harry Stack Sullivan, who acknowledged his debt to Mead, accepted Mead's belief that the self is not to be equated with individuality.[72] Sullivan felt that the uniqueness of self was an illusion. In his words, we have an "almost inescapable illusion that there is a perduring, unique, simple existent self, called variously 'me' or 'I,' and in some strange fashion, the patient's or the subject person's private property."[73] Inasmuch as the self is defined by others, individuals do not exist.

Many social scientists tend to recognize only the existence of a social self formed by a particular culture, whereas they deny or minimize the existence of a self generated from within. An exception is David Riesman, who understood that the interrelation between public and private selves forms the basis of certain character types.[74] In *The Lonely Crowd,* Riesman and his collaborators noted that American society after World War II underwent a gradual transformation that was reflected in an adaptive redistribution of character types—a transformation that might be described as a change in the ecology of personality.[75] Riesman believed that as societies evolve, there are concurrent changes in the structure of character. These changes follow a specified sequence from an original tradition-directed character type, to an inner-directed personality, and finally to an other-directed personality. Inner-directed individuals have an internal "gyroscope" that enables them to maintain a consistent sense of purposeful goal-directedness; they remain committed and aware of their moral values. I would characterize inner-directed individuals as people whose private self remains centered. Other-directed individuals are less centered, less certain of their goals and moral values and more dependent upon the signals they receive from others. This other-directedness, in my experience, is frequently accompanied by a relative or absolute alienation or dissociation from the private self. Riesman viewed other-directed people as socially adaptive, in that they are exceptionally sensitive to the wishes and actions of others. Riesman did not see the evolution of these different character types as sharply demarcated, but compared them to geological strata that are piled one on top of the other, with outcroppings of submerged types here and there. For example, he believed that among blacks and poor whites in the rural South of the United States, it is still possible to find remnants of the tradition-directed type.

I find Riesman's description to be an accurate prediction of a change in the ecology of the neuroses, for other-directedness has become one of the characteristic neuroses of our age. Patients today frequenty complain that they are unable to commit themselves either to a love relationship or to their work. This fear of commitment is sometimes accompanied by an inner sense of deadness and emptiness, a sense of futility, and the feeling that their lives lack meaning. Such patients believe that their lives are uncentered and lack purpose and direction. This form of neurosis is usually described as narcissistic, but it is also apparent that we are witnessing a proliferation of what Riesman called other-directed personalities. Compliance and sensitivity to the demands of others may be socially adaptive, but they are achieved at the expense of alienation from the private self. Such individuals remain uncommitted because they are out of touch with what is real and authentic within them, and hence do not know what they want. They have lost contact with that portion of the self that is creative and affectively alive.

This change in the relation between the private and public selves can also be inferred from literary sources. Lionel Trilling, in his celebrated book *Sincerity and Authenticity,* focuses on an earlier period, the late sixteenth and early seventeenth centuries.[76] For the individual who lived at that time, there was a greater congruence between the private self and the social self; indeed, this congruence was recognized as a virtue, the virtue of sincerity. (Trilling defines "sincerity" as the degree of congruence between feeling and avowal.) He suggests that something like a mutation in human nature occurred in the late sixteenth and early seventeenth centuries, when the distinction between public and private emerged: "One way of giving a synopsis of the whole complex psycho-historical occurrence is to say that the idea of society, much as we now conceive of it, came into being."[77]

It is interesting to consider the relations linking the psychological distinction between public and private selves and the degree of actual physical privacy afforded by the environment. We can observe in some patients that psychological intrusiveness is augmented when living conditions are such that one has no possibility of being by oneself. In the late sixteenth century, when, according to Trilling, a psychological distinction between private and public appeared, personal privacy in a physical sense hardly existed. Philippe Ariès informs us that until the end of the seventeenth century nobody was ever left alone.[78] The density of social life made isolation virtually impossible. People who shut themselves up in a room were looked upon as exceptional characters.

Goffman and the Multileveled Self

In *Other Times, Other Realities* I described the multiple levels of reality implicit in the self experience within the psychoanalytic setting. The psychoanalytic setting can be thought of as a frame that demarcates the reality contained within from the reality of ordinary life. This frame contains a "play" space within which illusions can flourish.

Erving Goffman had earlier proposed a very similar conception of a multileveled self, but I had not yet read his work. Goffman described a self that is defined in social interactions by means of a process of "framing" levels of reality.[79] He drew, as I had, upon the analogy to games; for in the playing of games in ordinary life, people have no problem moving from one level of reality to another. Goffman also viewed the interaction of self and others using another analogy, that of a theatrical performance: the part played by the individual is consciously and unconsciously tailored to the parts played by others in the audience, and the audience's response in turn influences the actor. Goffman's self is therefore a mask—not a mask that is entirely self created, but one that is mutually constructed. According to one interpretation, Goffman viewed the self as "a modern-day myth that people are forced to enact rather than a subjective entity that people privately possess."[80] He evidently did not believe in the existence of a private self that has coherence and continuity apart from the social stage. Goffman's self is a transient performance in which the individual aims to *control* the response of others.

Goffman's social self is an active agent: the individual projects an image of the self, which then influences the response of the other. Goffman's self is also more complex than the "Me" depicted by Mead. For Goffman, the self is an agency formed in social interaction, but it is not a "collective" entity simply formed by society, as Goffman's self is *intersubjectively* created: "I have said that when an individual appears before others his actions will influence the definition of the situation which they come to have. Sometimes he will intentionally and consciously express himself in a particular way, but chiefly because the tradition of his group or social status requires this kind of expression. The individual projects a definition of the situation when he appears before others, we must also see that the others, however passive their role may seem to be, will themselves effectively project a definition of the situation by virtue of their response."[81] Goffman believed that the participants, acting in concert, contribute to a single overall definition of the situation. Both individuals build up lines of responsive action. A social role will involve one or more parts, and the different parts may be presented at different times.

Goffman did not consider the self as a psychic structure, a fixed entity; he dwelt exclusively on the transient self, a Jamesian self of consciousness. It is a self that is multileveled, complex, and interactive. The idea of multiple levels, or different frames of reality created in interaction, should be distinguished from the structural concept of polarities within the self, such as the private and social self, and Kohut's bipolar self. We scarcely possess a language to describe this multileveled self, since this is an area that has been explored more extensively by novelists than by psychologists or social scientists. As Taylor has observed, *human life is irreducibly multileveled.*[82] Not only are there multiple levels of the self in relation to time, but there are also subtle adjustments of the self in every social interaction. We are never precisely the same person with different people. The self that emerges in social interaction is a constructed self. In Goffman's words, "The pre-established pattern of action which is unfolded during a performance and which may be presented or played through on other occasions may be called a 'part' or 'routine.' When the individual plays the same part to the same audience on different occasions a social relationship is likely to arise."[83]

Summary

In this chapter I have been guided by a Jamesian outline of the self, a tripartite notion consisting of, first, a bodily self; second, an aspect that James referred to as a "spiritual" self and that I call a "private" self; third, a social self. James's self is nearly coterminus with consciousness, but James was also aware of the structural aspect of self expressed as a continuing identity. Gerald Edelman's neurophysiological model of the biological self is likewise coterminus with consciousness. This biological self has evident survival value and rests upon structures of the nervous system that are different from those that mediate the perception of the external world. The continuity of the experience of the self is linked to the homeostatic function of the nervous system. The self is the repository of special value-laden memory systems.

One distinct adaptive advantage conferred upon those organisms who possess a sense of self is the ability to be free of the tyranny of ongoing events in real time. The experience of self enables the individual to model future actions by matching value-laden memories of past events with current perceptions. The ever-changing perceptions occurring in real time are recategorized via this matching with the memories of former states. Through a symbolic representation of the self, the organism is freed of the need to respond to any immediate perceptual stimuli. Edelman's biological self thus enables the individual to be relatively free of having to respond directly to environmental inputs. This biological conception of the self is diametrically opposed to the notion of a social self dependent upon inputs from the social environment.

In Edelman's model of the biological self, the sense of the continuity of the self amid the flux of perception is assured, since the self acts as a dominant template imposing order and coherence upon current perception. This suggests a resolution of the paradox of the continuity of the self amid the constant flux of consciousness.

Finally, Edelman's model of the biological self is a model based upon the evolution of individual differences. This contrasts with the now outdated evolutionary theory that Freud accepted, according to which the evolutionary process conferred adaptive advantages upon the group rather than the individual.

Systematic observations of infants suggest that the awareness of self appears early in infancy. Alongside the infant's need for relatedness is the infant's need for "private space." The infant can be "fueled" from within as well as from without. Researchers report that infants need time in which they are free to follow their own interests; disengagement has a place of equal importance with engagement. Being "fueled" from within leads to joy of mastery, a mastery that is self generating. This joy of mastery obviously extends into adult life; as Robert White observed, "seeking of efficacy is a primitive biological endowment."

These observations of infants support Winnicott's belief in a two-fold organization of the self: the true self and the false self. Winnicott's true self is the site of creative apperception of the world, as well as the locale in which contact is made with an inner world of impulse and feeling. Hence, the true self is the place of authenticity. If the true self becomes decentered and one loses contact with it, one also loses a sense of psychic aliveness.

The false self, as conceived by Winnicott, serves a defensive function. It originally serves to protect the infant's inner reality, and later functions as a means of preserving the privacy of the self. The false self is offered socially as an alternative self; there is no risk of exposure, since it is not "real." The private self, which supports an autonomy from the environment (the capacity to be alone), paradoxically requires, in early development, the protective, nonintrusive, continuing presence of the mother. Finally, Winnicott observed that there are aspects of the true self which remain forever private and are never communicated to others.

Kohut's theory of the self is essentially that of a social self; there is no recognition of "fueling" from within, nor is there recognition of the importance of noncommunication. That is to say, Kohut's self psychology recognizes only states of relatedness. His theory is that of a self whose integrity and cohesion are dependent on the selfobject in the same way "the body is dependent upon oxygen."

I consider Kohut's most original contribution to be his radical stance with regard to the self/ego dilemma. Like William James, Kohut believed that the subjective experience of the self required no further objectification. He could be described as a radical phenomenologist whose theory of the self is, as near as possible, congruent with the subject's self experience. But this stance behind the primacy of the individual's subjective experience also reveals the limitations of phenomenology and self psychology. This can be seen in self psychology's silence with regard to some experiences of great psychological significance, such as object loss. In Kohut's view, such a topic belongs within the realm of biology, within the world of "extrospection."

The process of thinking about the self can be viewed as a subtext of all of Western philosophy. The idea of a private self, known only to its possessor and perhaps also to an omniscient God, is a very ancient concept. The ancients recognized that commitment to a private morality enabled the individual to be free of a tyrannical environment. The modern idea of a private self can be traced to Saint Augustine, who viewed this inner self as a source not only of moral values but also of authenticity.

In certain sociological traditions, this private self is minimized in favor of a self that owes its existence to the other. This is essentially the view of George Herbert Mead, who believed that only when the self is treated as an object by others can one discover one's own self. The self is formed as a consequence of socially bestowed "roles"—is formed as a "generalized" other.

A different sociological tradition is represented by the work of David Riesman and his collaborators. Riesman suggested that as societies evolve, there are concurrent changes in character structure: from an originally tradition-directed personality, to an inner-directed personality, and finally to an other-directed personality. I understand Riesman to be describing the establishment of a private self, followed by a gradual decentering of the private self. His analysis corresponds to an observable change in the ecology of the neurosis. The notion of the so-called narcissistic personality, who is overly dependent on social affirmation, corresponds very well with Riesman's concept of the other-directed personality. These are individuals who may be socially adaptive in that they obtain their cues from others, but they have lost touch with their inner core to such an extent that they remain uncommitted both in their love relationships and in their work.

Still another sociological tradition regarding the self is represented by the work of Erving Goffman. Like Mead, Goffman described a self derived from social interactions. But it seems to me that Goffman's account is more sophisticated than Mead's in that it incorporates the multiple realities present in social interactions. Furthermore, Goffman emphasized that the self is an active agent: individuals project an image, which in turn influences the behavior of the other. Goffman's account is consistent with theories that view self formation as an intersubjective process.

3

The Private Self in
Public Space

> We must reserve a little back-shop, all our own, entirely free,
> wherein to establish our true liberty and principal retreat and
> solitude.
>
> MONTAIGNE, *Essays,* tr. E. S. Trechmann

Let us now look at the various defensive means that individuals use to protect the private self from intrusion. We
shall see that the private self is the locus of personal value
and personal meaning, and that there is a high psychic pay-
ment exacted when there is a decentering or a loss of contact
with this private self.

Most experienced psychoanalytic clinicians would not
question the existence of a private self, for their patients
teach them that there is an inner core of the self that must be
protected from intrusion. It can be argued that this is merely
a sign of psychopathology, an indication that a particular patient suffers from a sense of self that is vulnerable and fragile. Although this is undoubtedly true, it would be a mistake
to separate psychopathology and health so sharply. Psychopathology simply illuminates by exaggeration that which is
present in all of us. I would suggest that the need to protect
the private self from intrusions by others is universal.

The idea of claiming one's own psychological space is an
idea that is well established in folk psychology. There appears to be natural progression from the concepts of folk

psychology to the scientific use of such concepts. George Lakoff has shown how abstract psychological concepts can arise from images related to the body.[1] This would be a natural extension of the idea that even as our bodies occupy physical space, our minds occupy psychological space. A mental space is a site for conceptualization and thought.[2] One often hears patients complain that their partner intrudes into their "space" or does not allow them "space." The need for psychological space, the need for time-out from relatedness, has been noted as early as infancy. Recall Sander's observation that infants require time for "open space"; they need to be disengaged from the mother in order to develop their own focus of attention and personal interests. The psychoanalysis of adults gives credence to Sander's statement that disengagement has a place of equal importance with engagement. Kohut likened the need for affirming selfobjects to the need for oxygen; but it could also be said that one cannot remain psychologically alive without private space. If one lives within a family that does not respect the need for private space, one can experience this as a suffocation of the self, a denial of personhood, a form of "soul murder." There is a relation between psychological space and actual physical privacy. Private space can exist in the absence of physical privacy, and, conversely, private space can be encroached upon even if there is physical privacy.[3]

Private space opens when one is disengaged from others. But there is more to private space than simple nonrelatedness. For private space is experienced as an extension of the self: private space means that this space is *mine*—it is not neutral territory or space shared with others. William James noted this relationship between the self and what is *mine*.[4] What I include as part of my self is subject to both expansion and contraction; what is mine may contract if an individual disowns what he is or what he has; or what is mine can extend to include an identification not only with my thoughts but with my spouse, children, possessions, and so on. In analogous fashion, private space can expand and contract in accordance with the needs and functions of the private self at any given moment in time. Private space can function as an alternative environment.

Freud, too, recognized that the self can be an alternative source of gratification. In depicting the methods that people employ to find happiness, Freud said: "There is no golden rule which applies to everyone: every man must find out for himself in what particular fashion he can be saved. The man who is predominately erotic will give first preference to his emotional relationships to other people; the narcissistic man, who inclines to be self-sufficient, will seek his main satisfaction in his internal mental processes."[5] The term "narcissistic" in this context is misleading, for Freud himself would have to be counted among those who find their main source of satisfaction in their own mental processes.

The creation of alternative worlds is not the privilege of the artist alone. For those whose actual world is abhorrent, this capacity to create an alternative inner world may be the only means of self preservation. This view of the self is consistent with Edelman's notion of the biological self. In Edelman's view, one function of the self is to provide a coherent schema of past, present, and future that effectively removes the individual from the inputs of real time. That is to say, the biological self enables one to be relatively autonomous from current time.

The autonomy of the self rests upon the paradoxical fact that this autonomy must initially be provided for by another. Winnicott observed that "time is kept going by the mother."[6] The creation of a substitute inner world initially requires a sense of continuity that is provided for by the continued presence of the real or imagined object. This is Winnicott's paradox: the child's creative use of solitude requires the presence of the mother in order to affirm the continuity of the self. If one is entirely enclosed within the self, one begins to doubt the reality of one's constructions, so that some measure of affirmation is needed not only to preserve the continuity of the self but also to preserve one's sense of reality. Psychotics, too, can be said to live within a personal world that they have substituted for external reality. But the essential difference is that in the case of the psychotic, the facilitating object is no longer present.

The private self is thus a paradoxical structure that frees one from dependency, yet requires the other for its continued existence. This paradox is clearly illustrated in disorders of the self, such as the so-called schizoid personality, where defenses are clearly directed toward the preservation of private space. Although the schizoid person can be said to live within his or her private space, the autonomy of the self is more apparent than real, in that the self is experienced as extremely fragile and vulnerable to the responses of the other. The following vignette shows this clearly.

A particular patient of mine was suffering from a disorder of the self, but was definitely not schizophrenic or in any sense psychotic. This is the woman I referred to in Chapter 1 who believed, as a child, that the octopus used its tentacles to suck out the contents of its victims.[7] She felt that to be in the presence of another person exposed her to a similar risk, and thus she feared that the continued existence of her self was held hostage to the response of others. Her sense of self was not threatened when she was alone, however.

My patient believed that the core of her self could be connected to another unknown self by some secret passage. It was as if her present self occupied a *known* universe but a future self could occupy a different *unknown* universe. She visualized this concretely as a self occupying a sphere that was connected by a mysterious or hidden passage to this other, unknown sphere. When in the presence of another person, her known self was at risk, in that it could be drained into the unknown sphere. She thus could be transformed into a different person. (Recall the similar anxiety that terrified William James, who, during a period of depression, felt that he might lose his own self and become transformed into a hideous alien self, similar to an idiotic epileptic youth he once saw in an asylum.)

My patient referred to her private self as a "core," which she could control by "popping" it in or out. She could "pop out" this core to preserve her private self from intrusion or humiliation. When her core was "popped out," what remained was a "false self" which she believed to be thin, stiff, and shallow, because it was lacking in authentic affects. Fairbairn observed that by playing a role, schizoid individuals may be able to express feeling and make what appears to be impressive social contact; but since they are playing a part, they can disown it and thus preserve their own inner personality.[8] My patient was aware, however, that when the core of her personality was absent, social contact was not quite adequate: she appeared to other people as distant and flat. She "resided," so to speak, within this core, and without it she was not truly there. If the core was breached, it felt as if she were being raped or as if someone were breaking into her house. "Popping out" this core was analogous to removing her valuables to a safer place.

This core of the self, if breached by another person, became vulnerable to the pain of humiliation, which she felt to be nearly unbearable. My patient believed that in a sense she could be psychically "raped." But the orifice through which this rape could occur was not the genitals but the eyes. It is through one's eyes that one makes social contact; the eyes are the guardian of the soul. One glimpses the soul through the eyes, since the expression of the eyes reveals authentic affective states which can otherwise be masked by the face. My patient therefore had great difficulty letting others look into her eyes, and generally averted her glance. The prospect of an ophthalmic examination sent her into a panic. Yet she liked observing other people's eyes, to obtain knowledge of their psychic states—whether, for example, they held their gaze and were psychically present or were shifty-eyed and psychically absent. She classified people according to whether they had "good" or "bad" eyes. The eyes were, for her, an early warning system.

After a period of psychotherapy, she started a psychoanalysis. When we shifted her treatment, so as to use the couch instead of talking face to face, she felt—to our mutual surprise—much more comfortable on the couch, since I could not see her eyes and she was relieved of the burden of having to read my eyes. "What do you fear the other person will see in your eyes?" I asked her. She responded that the other person would look into her eyes and see chaos—a revelation that would be unbearably humiliating. It would be as if a defect of the self were being exposed, as if she were, say, hiding a tail. To be humiliated by others meant that she was being controlled by them and that she could be infinitely exploited. She associated to the abuses practiced by leaders of cults, feeling that such abuses were akin to the control of a subject by a hypnotist.

Whenever she was caught off guard, whenever something unexpected happened, she was unable to regulate the ideal distance from others. Her sense of self was thus vulnerable not only to the unempathic response of others but simply to the act of becoming known to others. And her own connection to others also placed her self in jeopardy. For example, when she felt an empathic connection with another person, she felt merged with that person. And if she felt merged, she then feared that she would lose her sense of self. She experienced her sense of self as if she were a still camera whose shutter clicked intermittently. Her sense of self was intermittent, rather than continuous as in a movie camera. Merging with another threatened her sense of the intactness and continuity of the self.

Authenticity and the Private Self

The fundamental rule of psychoanalysis enjoins the analysand to say everything that comes to mind without deciding what is relevant or irrelevant. For many patients this is an impossible injunction, because it threatens the very survival of the private self. Some patients apparently comply with this injunction and fill the hours with talk. But if the talk is delivered in an unvarying monotone, if it is talk from which the affective charge has been removed, the analyst may feel lost in a sea of words. In the absence of authenticity, there can be no psychoanalytic dialogue; meaning cannot be communicated without some trace of genuine feeling. In some cases intense feelings appear to be communicated, but the analyst may find later that the affects are inauthentic—are exaggerated or false. To communicate genuine feeling is also an expression of need, so that the communication of authentic affects is intrinsically object seeking.[9] The converse is also true: the noncommunication of affect is a communication of self sufficiency.

The analyst's empathic understanding of the patient is dependent upon the affective metacommunications that accompany the patient's words.[10] The patient's affects are contagious and excite the analyst's own affective responses. In the absence of these contagious affects, the analyst is deprived of empathic tools. Sometimes the only way an analyst can infer sadness is by actually seeing the patient's tears.

If affects are object seeking, the communication of authentic feelings will destroy the illusion of self sufficiency. It must be understood that the decision not to communicate affect is not a conscious decision; it is an unconscious defense similar to the automatic defenses that the body employs. It is a defense employed with the aim of preserving one's private self and private space.[11] In addition to this motive of preserving the private self, individuals may avoid communicating genuine feeling because they are so distant from their private self that they themselves are unaware of what they are feeling. This has been described as "alienation" from the self,[12] or, as I call it, "decentering" of the self.

If patients are completely walled off within their private space, this invariably induces a counteraffective response in the analyst.[13] Analysts feel that such patients are not in the room with them. When I am with such a person I find myself becoming bored or sleepy, or at times angry at being excluded. It is impossible for me not to respond, when I am in the continued presence of another human being who does not relate to me. This is not a question of the patient's being uncooperative or defiant, but is an indication of the automatic defensive measures introduced in order to preserve private space. When patients are encased within their private self, their endopsychic experience is that of being in a cocoon or a plastic bubble. This may be a wonderfully safe retreat, or a prison from which there is no escape, in accordance with the intrinsically paradoxical autonomous and dependent nature of the self.

I have described this state of affairs, which characterizes the opening phase of many analyses (a phase that may last several years), as a sphere within a sphere.[14] This experience of being within one's own world yet encased in the larger world is not limited to psychoanalytic therapy. As John Hull indicates in his autobiography, he, too, came to experience his blindness as a sphere within a sphere: "Blindness is a little world, authentic and integrated of itself, and yet surrounded by and held within a greater world, the world of the sighted."[15] I interpret this statement as an affirmation that the private self can be held by others. As I have indicated, I believe this to be an important aspect of the psychotherapeutic process.

The continuity of the self is assured by the holding function of the psychoanalytic or psychotherapeutic setting; at the same time, patients are encased within their own private space. The therapeutic setting is the larger sphere in which the smaller sphere of the private self is held incommunicado. In terms of the therapeutic process, this state of affairs is truly paradoxical: if a patient is not communicating, the therapist experiences this as a resistance, but it is a resistance that proves to be therapeutic. For within this state of noncommunication and nonrelatedness, the patient is reestablishing contact with his or her private self. For some, it is their first opportunity to experience their own thoughts within a protected environment.[16] Accordingly, therapists may be surprised to observe that clinical improvement has occurred without any specific interventions on their part; in fact, it is the absence of intrusive interventions in itself that facilitates therapeutic change.[17] Therapists note progress when their patients appear to be increasingly there, to be more present, to be more in the room with them. With the increasing communication of genuine affects, patients seem more psychically alive, and in this sense more human. As patients gradually come into better contact with their own authentic affective core, they feel that their private self is more secure and are then able to allow their private space to become more permeable to others.

I do not plan to discuss the theory of this therapeutic action in detail, since I have done so elsewhere.[18] Suffice it to say that therapeutic action is multileveled and relies on the safety that is provided by the continuity and reliability of the therapeutic setting, as well as the process in which the patient's affective experiences are recategorized and brought within the hegemony of the self.

Freud's famous aphorism "Wo Es war, soll Ich werden" was translated by Strachey as "Where id was there shall ego be."[19] Lacan rendered this more accurately as "Where *it* was there shall *I* be."[20] When things are viewed in this light, one aim of psychoanalytic treatment is to extend the domain of the personal over the impersonal, to extend the domain of self over the impersonal *it.*

Freud viewed *das Es,* the *it* (or *id*), as a reservoir of impersonal instincts. When the *it* becomes the *I,* the affects derived from these impulses and desires become personal affects. The infant, as Winnicott says, rediscovers the *personal* impulse: "The individual who has developed the capacity to be alone is constantly able to rediscover the personal impulse, and the personal impulse is not wasted because the state of being alone is something which (though paradoxically) always implies that someone else is there."[21] Feelings and impulses are experienced as intrusions if they are felt to originate from an area outside private space, as if such impulses were part of an external environment.[22] It is the centering of affects within the self that leads to a sense of psychic aliveness. R. D. Laing, too, spoke of affective centering as that which enables the individual to feel real and alive, to feel that he or she is an entity with continuity in time and existence in space.[23]

If we speak of decentering and alienation of the self, we assume a self that has at some earlier time been more centered. As we noted earlier, such centering of the self is facilitated through a process of maternal attunement.[24] The mother who is able to match her infant's affects also enables that infant to process its own affects. Research on infants appears to confirm W. R. Bion's theory of the container and the contained.[25] According to Bion, the mother enables her infant to "digest" anxiety because she contains and then, in a sense, metabolizes it for the child, returning the anxiety to the child in a less toxic form, very much as a mother bird will predigest her baby's food. If this process succeeds, the child can then say, "These are *my* feelings." The infant seems able, cognitively, to differentiate self from other quite early, but inasmuch as there is a synchrony of affective states in the mother and child, uncertainty as to whose affects are being experienced may continue into adult life. Since affects are intrinsically uncontrollable, people sometimes feel that affects do not belong to them (see Chapter 7).

The Decentering of the Private Self

If one aim of psychoanalytic treatment is to enlarge and extend the domain of the personal, a question naturally arises: How did the self become alienated from itself? There is a widely held assumption, supported by direct observation of infants,[26] that the self is originally a holistic gestalt. Psychoanalytic observation suggests a similar view—namely, that a lack of cohesion of the self is indicative of psychopathology. Recall Fairbairn's account of how the self responds to traumatic interactions with caretakers by replicating within the self an internalized object relationship, which then becomes dissociated from the central ego (self). Also recall Winnicott's view: that the false self protects the child's psychic reality from noxious intrusions, and that behind the false self lies a true self waiting to be found.

Likewise, it is common knowledge that young children frequently lose their spontaneity and creativity as they become older. That is to say, they lose their sense of authenticity, which means either that they have become decentered from their inner self or that their creativity has become entirely private and is no longer communicated.

A skeptical observer may counter: Mightn't the belief in an originally authentic self from which one becomes estranged be nothing more than an idealized, mythic interpretation of a lost childhood? When my patients declare that they are empty and have nothing inside them, they also remain skeptical when I state that they really do possess an authentic self waiting to be found. My confidence in this assertion rests on the knowledge that most patients will establish better contact with their private self in the course of psychoanalytic treatment. If there were no previously existing authentic self, it would be impossible to expect that the therapeutic process could restore it.

When the child's private space is habitually violated, vital defenses are erected. But the defenses used against the intruder are, unfortunately, turned upon the self as well. In accordance with Fairbairn's principle that traumatic relationships between the self and others are recreated within the self, *the means employed to protect private space against intrusion by others are also recreated within the self.* Individuals become estranged from their own affective core, and are as false and inauthentic within themselves as they are with others. In the struggle to preserve private space, they therefore achieve only a pyrrhic victory. Ironically, the fight to protect the private self continues even after the individual has lost contact with it. It is as if a householder were to maintain a burglar alarm long after misplacing her jewels. *In closing oneself off from others, one inadvertently closes oneself off from the self.*

Mikhail Bakhtin (1895–1975), a Russian author who has been described as both a "philosopher of human science" and a "theoretician of literature," has beautifully captured this process of the interrelationship between private self and social self:

I achieve self-consciousness, I become myself only by revealing myself to another, through another and with another's help. The most important acts, constitutive of self-consciousness, are determined by their relation to another consciousness ("a thou"). *Cutting oneself off, isolating oneself, closing oneself off, those are the basic reasons for loss of self*... It turns out that every internal experience occurs on the border, it comes across another, and this essence resides in this intense encounter... The very being of man (both internal and external) is a *profound communication. To be means to communicate*... To be means to be for the other, and through him, for oneself. Man has no internal sovereign territory; he is all and always on the boundary; looking within himself, he looks *in the eyes of the other or through the eyes of the other*... I cannot do without the other; I cannot become myself without the other; I must find myself in the other, finding the other in me (in mutual reflection and perception). Justification cannot be justification of *oneself,* confession cannot be confession of *oneself.* I receive my name from the other, and this name exists for the other (to name oneself is to engage in usurpation).[27]

The Private Self Preserved: Generating Private Space

George Orwell is reported to have said that at fifty everyone has the face he deserves.[28] Behind this witticism there is a biological truth: in a certain sense, we create ourselves. We are in part responsible for our face, and we are also to some extent responsible for our brain. As we have seen, the brain develops as a structure that is tailored to the life experience of each human being.[29] The remarkable range of individual variation in the morphology of the central nervous system exceeds genetic constraints and is attributable to the functional activities that occur in development at every level, from the cell upward. This is to assert not that an element of some mystical *will* enters into ontogeny but that the development of the brain reflects both a structural and a functional individuality. In a literal sense, we create ourselves.

If it is a fact, as Winnicott believed, that the infant, through the spontaneous gesture, is creative at birth, infancy can also be said to mark the onset of the creation of a private self. Winnicott believed that if the mother responds with sensitivity to the infant's desire, this reinforces in the infant a sense of beneficent omnipotence. Some vestiges of this primordial grandiosity remain in most people, and form the basis for a healthy faith in the self. On the other hand, we also know from the analysis of adults that when there is a significant failure in the parental holding environment, reliance on a grandiose self may substitute for an absence of parental holding and the outcome may not prove to be so benevolent.[30] In this case the omnipotent self is formed as a compensation for the absence of safety in the external world; the private self becomes an alternative holding environment, affording magical protection. In the psychoanalysis of some individuals who could be described as suffering from a narcissistic personality disorder, the analyst may frequently observe aspects of this grandiose self. For example, one of my patients, as a latency-aged child, believed himself to be Superman and thought that with sufficient practice he could teach himself to fly—that if he wished hard enough, anything could happen. Confrontation with the reality principle was brushed aside, since he was convinced that if he could not fly now it would happen some time in the *future*. As an adult, he continued to assume that anything was possible if he desired it with sufficient intensity. Another patient of mine had a birthmark on her buttock that was shaped like Australia; she believed that this fact endowed her with secret powers that were commensurate with the size of that continent. This fantasy of the self was revealed with great reluctance, and only after a very trusting patient-analyst relationship had been established.

In these instances, reliance on the powers of a magical omnipotent self appeared to be necessary for the patients' psychic survival, because there were no other means of protection. To expose this private self to others, therefore, was to endanger their safety in the world. Such people, understandably, experience their private self as extremely fragile and vulnerable.

One may speak of the shadow of the object falling upon the ego, but it must be emphasized that the object, too, is only a shadow. For what is internalized does not correspond only to that which the individual has experienced. Children internalize more than their parents' "objective" behavior, values, and attitudes. Freud noted that children's superegos do not correspond to the severity of treatment they have experienced, since a child who has been treated leniently may acquire a very strict conscience.[31] We also know that children, not uncommonly, defend against an identification with a parent by choosing attitudes and values diametrically opposed to those of the parent. Such counteridentifications are self created. With the development of the child's capacity for symbolization and imaginary play, experience itself can be transformed. The objects with which the child identifies may originate as "actual" persons but are then transformed into subjectively created persons.

The structure of the self thus contains affective memories of actual relationships, interspersed with fantasy. In this blending process it is not only the *child's* fantasies that are internalized: the child also internalizes the *parent's* fantasies of the child. To these fantasies are added various misidentifications of the child with the parent's self and other internalized objects that are part of the parent's history.[32]

In addition to our parents, we also identify with idealized persons, who may be actual persons but who exist for us only in our imagination. We create ourselves by identifying with those persons that we wish to become. The possibilities here are endless. For many people this is a bootstrapping operation that lifts them out of the world into which they have been born. There is evidently a wild card or joker in the pack of psychic development. For some, the identification is not so much with a particular person as with the ideas that that person represents. Such identifications can become the source of sustained lifelong motivation and moral values. I use the term "moral values" to refer not only to ethical values but also to all that the individual believes to be "good." Such self-created identifications can be said to expand the area of private space.

The idealized persons from which such interests derive may replace and offset identifications with the actual parents. The values and attitudes thus internalized may form the nexus of counteridentifications that support individuation. In this way, individuals create their own private morality. There is, within the self, an ideal self that must be distinguished from Freud's relatively impersonal superego, which enforces a shared or group morality. Iris Murdoch has referred to this process as the individual's quest for the *good,* a quest for perfectibility.[33] Murdoch argues for the existence of a private language that reflects the historicity of the self. She questions Wittgenstein's assertion that private languages are an impossibility.

Not all people, of course, bootstrap themselves in this fashion; there are apples that do not fall very far from the tree. The extent to which one differentiates oneself from parental identifications and separates oneself from the nuclear family evidently depends on multiple factors, the most obvious of which is the nature of one's innate endowment. We all know that within a given family there may be siblings whose lives take a quantum leap out of their original social, cultural, and economic milieu, leaving behind other siblings whose identity, values, and achievements remain in the more expectable range.[34] I have identified "separation guilt" as another factor, apart from innate endowment, that may determine the extent to which individuals can differentiate themselves from the nuclear family.[35] People who bootstrap themselves out of the family milieu frequently develop an intense sense of guilt. Such people believe that they do not have the right to a (separate) life. Many of my patients have expressed the fantasy that as they become separate from the parent (usually of the same sex), that parent may become damaged. In extreme cases, patients reveal the fantasy that to become separate will kill the parent. In less extreme forms of the fantasy, patients believe that to become an autonomous person is a form of disloyalty. Therefore, some choose not to expose their individuality to others; but in the process, they may lose contact with and come to distrust their own inner source of creativity.

The road to individuation is undoubtedly made easier if one can find sustenance in the values contained within the private self. As Abraham Maslow reported, "Self-actualizing people are, without one single exception, involved in a cause outside their own skin, in something outside of themselves. They are devoted, working at something, something which is very precious to them—some calling or vocation in the old sense, the priestly sense. They are working at something which fate has called them to somehow and which they work at and which they love."[36]

Likewise, those who can find sources of sustenance within the private self tend to be more resilient to the blows of fate. James Anthony and Bertram Cohler observed a number of children who survived intensely traumatic environments. One such child who was subjected to the psychotic outbursts of a manic-depressive mother remained composed amid the mother's attacks and thrived both scholastically and interpersonally. She was asked to make a cardboard construction of what it felt like to live with her sick mother. She constructed a "castle," which she described as "the little space that she arranged for herself in the household and into which she could retreat when things got rough."[37]

The biographies of many self-actualizing individuals who survived horrendous childhoods attest to the creation of similar "castles." This is especially clear in the biographies of great artists who survived by means of their creativity. For some, this creative transformation of reality is the means of psychic survival. One thinks, for example, of Charlie Chaplin, whose father deserted the family and whose schizophrenic mother was periodically hospitalized. At these times, Chaplin and his older brother were domiciled in public institutions for the poor. When their mother recovered, there would be a joyous family reunion.[38] There is a famous scene in *City Lights* where the Little Tramp meets a millionaire, who when drunk is his best friend. He brings the Tramp home and entertains him lavishly. But when the millionaire becomes sober, he no longer recognizes the Tramp and throws him out of his house. This scene suggests a parody of Chaplin's relationship to his mother, who was by turns totally loving and totally absent. In *Soul Murder,* Leonard Shengold describes Rudyard Kipling's horrific childhood.[39] Kipling and his sister, for some unknown reason, were abandoned by their parents for a period of six years and placed in the care of a married couple, who acted as foster parents. The wife and her sadistic older son tyrannized Kipling and his sister. The two children were at times forbidden to speak to each other, and Kipling was severely beaten and humiliated for what was termed "lying." Shengold suggests that Kipling wrote as a means of revenging himself and finding an outlet for his enormous rage. Ingmar Bergman, in his own autobiography, likewise describes being beaten and humiliated for lying.[40] In his case, the punishment was inflicted by his father. In addition to being beaten, Bergman, who had an intense fear of the dark, was locked inside a special cupboard and was told that inside this cupboard lived an animal that ate the toes of little children. Bergman survived this horror by hiding a flashlight in the cupboard and pretending that he was at the cinema. Later he actually acquired a magic lantern, a toy movie projector, which allowed him to create an alternative make-believe world, an endeavor that became his life's work.

But survival through the expansion of the private self is not limited to those with artistic talent. There are many individuals who survive in unsupportive environments by means of daydreams and fantasies. For example, I once had a patient who believed (I think correctly) that her mother truly hated her. Her father, who was incapacitated because of organic brain disease, was unavailable to her. She therefore created an alternative environment of complex daydreams and fantasies, a reality that paralleled and constantly accompanied her other activities in the real world. Her consciousness was in this fashion split, and she could effectively live within these two separate levels of reality.

John Hull, who became blind in middle age, relates how he recreated himself after completing the process of mourning for his lost eyesight: "There has been a strange change in the state or the kind of activity in my brain. It seems to have turned in upon itself to find inner resources. Being denied the stimulus of much of the outside world, it has had to sort out its own functions and priorities. I now feel clearer, more excited and more adventurous intellectually than ever before in my life. I find myself connecting more, remembering more, making more links in my mind between various things I have read. Sometimes I come home in the evening and feel that my mind is almost bursting with new ideas and new horizons."[41]

We have long known that there is no simple relationship between environmental trauma and psychopathology. I am suggesting that those individuals who have access to their private self can create an alternative internal environment that enlarges the domain of the personal so that they can transcend the experiences of real time.

Summary

As Stephen Toulmin has pointed out, there was a time in the history of philosophy when empiricists accepted the notion that inner experience is always private.[42] Privacy in this context might be called a "logical" privacy, in that one cannot fully share with another the data of one's senses.[43] But the idea of private space suggests something different. It refers to one's experience while one is in a state of nonrelatedness, and this experience is private because it is not communicated (though of course it may be communicated at some future time). It is experience that is claimed as *mine* alone. These periods of nonrelatedness, I suggest, are as necessary and as vital as states of relatedness. For individuals who must cope with dreadful environments, private space can be the place in which alternative worlds are created, worlds that guarantee psychic survival.

The schizoid defense of noncommunication can be viewed as a means of protecting private space. The deepest anxiety experienced in such cases is that intrusion into one's private space will disrupt continuity of the sense of self. The strength of the private self safeguards private space. This strength, in turn, depends upon one's remaining in contact with an affective core. The integrity of this affective core can be disrupted and decentered in a variety of ways. One familiar source of disruption can be traced to disturbances in the mother-child relationship that result in a relative impairment of affect attunement and affect regulation. Another source lies in the fact that the means employed to protect private space from intrusion are recreated within the self. In closing oneself off from others, one may inadvertently close oneself off from oneself.

The successful preservation of the private self can be seen in the biographies of certain artists who have used their art to transform the miseries of their childhood. The creative imagination essentially translates traumatic experiences into the language of the private self, and thus ensures the continuity and preservation of the self. One affirms the self through the creation of meaning.

4

The Dialectic of Self and Other

All of me, why not take all of me?
S. SIMONS AND G. MARKS; sung by Billie Holiday

Consideration of the private self in the presence of others, in public space, is implicitly an appraisal of the self and the other functioning as an ensemble, as an intersubjective system. In the previous chapter I examined the need to preserve private space from the danger of intrusion. I would now like to narrow the focus and consider not the danger of intrusion but the problem of dependency, from which fresh conflicts and dangers may arise.

Let us look at two attributes of this intersubjective system. The first is the extension of the self into the other, or of the other into the self: the degree to which the self is experienced as part of the other. We might speak of this, conversely, as the degree to which the other is experienced as separate, external, and alien. Superimposed on this aspect is a different dimension: that of desire, power, and control. This will lead us to consider the relative proportions of altruism and self interest, and the inequality of need and desire, which makes one partner more vulnerable than the other. It will be a consideration of the symmetry and *asymmetry* of self and other. The wish to merge with another is invariably accompanied by an overidealization of the other, a form of loving. And, as we shall see, the perception of the other as absolutely alien and separate is invariably accompanied by some form of hatred.

The attributes of self and other that we choose to focus on no doubt reflect certain values embedded in Western culture which found their expression in philosophy long before that discipline became differentiated from psychology. The theme of love as a union with the other can be found in Plato's myth concerning the origin of sexual love, a myth described in the *Symposium.* Hegel, with his parable of the master/slave relationship, asserts in *The Phenomenology of Mind* that there is no consciousness of self without consciousness of the other. I doubt whether our present psychology of intersubjectivity could have developed without Hegel.[1] For Hegel appeared to have intuitively grasped the fundamental aspects of the psychology of self and other.

According to Plato, we all seek to lose our separateness. This primordial need to merge with another utilizes erotic love but is more fundamental than eroticism. In the *Symposium,* Plato has Aristophanes recount an ancient myth that answers the question: What is the nature of love?[2] Aristophanes describes how human beings were originally spherical, with four legs, four arms, two sets of genitals, and two identical faces set upon a single head but looking in opposite directions. In the beginning, there were three sexes: male, female, and an androgynous or hermaphroditic sex consisting of a male half and a female half. But Zeus split them all, like apples that are halved for pickling. Each human being, having been separated in this fashion and having only one side, like a flat fish, is always looking for his or her other half. Those descended from the spherical male seek sexual union with males, those descended from the primeval woman seek union with females, and those descended from the asymmetrical androgynous sex seek union in heterosexual love. Aristophanes relates that Hephaestus, the lame smithy god, asked a couple who were lying side by side, "What do you people want of each other? Do you desire to be wholly one? If this is what you desire I am ready to melt you into one and let you grow together, so that being two you shall become one." Everyone who heard this proposal agreed that melting into each other, becoming one instead of two, was the expression of their ancient need.

Hegel can justifiably be termed the first intersubjective or relational psychologist.[3] In his chapter "Lordship and Bondage" in *The Phenomenology of Mind,* he described the interrelationship between one's own consciousness of self and another person's consciousness of self.[4] Consciousness of self exists only when acknowledged by the other. Hegel posited a reciprocal formation of two consciousnesses: there can be no master without a slave, and no slave without a master. This is true for both parties: the self is mirrored in the other, and the other is mirrored in the self; they require each other for substantiation. Hegel therefore considered self and other simultaneously, as an ensemble. He viewed self and other in a symmetrical mirror relationship, as well as in an asymmetrical relationship of dependency, desire, and control. But, Hegel reasoned, if the self is only the mirror of the other, then the unique and distinctive traits of the self, those things that constitute individuality and personhood, are obliterated. Hegel thereby identified a profound human dilemma, for if the self is defined by means of its reflection in the other, it loses its personhood. Therefore, in order to define oneself, one must create externality by negating the existence of the other, ultimately by killing the other as something that is alien and foreign to the self. But the killing of the other is not to be taken literally, for if the killing is actual the parable would be over.[5] (In a similar fashion, Winnicott would later say that the externality of the other is established through hatred, but it is essential that both parties survive.)[6]

Hegel recognized that self and other exist in a dialectical relationship that is fundamentally paradoxical, causing dilemmas for which there is no ultimate solution. The simultaneous dependency and autonomy of the self that Hegel portrayed is the paradox with which we have become familiar as the paradox of the private and social selves. He was also aware of the paradox of the self as a fixed identity within the flux of experience. As a consequence of the dilemmas generated by these multiple paradoxes, Hegel believed that the self becomes divided against itself. Hegel therefore can be said to have recognized the concept of the splitting of the self. Taylor, in his exegesis of Hegel's *Phenomenology of Mind,* writes: "What we have is an oscillation between a sense of our own self-identity, and an equally acute sense of our dependence on a changing, shifting external reality. The subject has to accept the fact of an inner division, in which the inner self is painfully divided, into an ideal immutable and self-identical being on one side and plunged in a world of confusion and change on the other."[7]

For Hegel, the asymmetry of self and other results from the asymmetry of desire, which leads to the possibility of control and domination by an other who is free of desire. The master is the one who is independent and self sufficient (exists only for himself); the slave is the one whose entire existence is for the other.[8] In order to reestablish personhood, it is necessary to negate and ultimately extinguish the other. But both master and slave engage in a dialectical process: the master cannot exist without the slave, for if the master is complete within himself he cannot learn from the world.

Although Hegel does not speak of omnipotence, he is essentially describing the condition of Lordship as a state of exalted isolation that accompanies a belief in one's omnipotence. *"The master is the consciousness that exists [only] for itself."*[9] The master is completely sufficient unto himself and without desire for the other. It is desire, therefore, that makes one a slave. The omnipotent master rejects all that is foreign; he rejects that which is perceived as the nonself. He therefore wishes to negate the individuality of the other and reduce the other to a "thing." "In thought I am free, because I am not in another, but remain quite within my own purview."[10] By not acknowledging the existence of the other, the master is not limited or constricted by others. But inasmuch as knowledge and truth are intersubjective, the omnipotent master does not learn from experience; he is deprived of the capacity to learn from others. "Each is indeed certain of its own self, but not of the other, and hence its own certainty of itself is without truth. For its truth would be merely that of its own individual existence."[11] Here, the slave who is attached to the other has an advantage over the master and gradually transcends his inferior position. The slave, unlike the master, learns from experience. The slave ultimately transcends his condition, because he has to struggle in order to achieve mastery. In his description of the omnipotent master in splendid isolation, and of the dependent yet engaged slave, Hegel describes an essential aspect of the human condition, an oscillation between engagement and disengagement, between solitude and relatedness. It is also evident that Hegel's dialectic of slave and master not only is an attribute of self and an *external* other, but refers to the *internalized* relation of the idealized self to the actual self. Freud would later describe such divisions as being between the ego and the ideal self (ego ideal). The self may be diminished and held in thrall by the ideal self, whose goals can never be reached.

In a few tightly written pages, Hegel anticipated many fundamental aspects of the psychology of the self. First, he anticipated the psychology of mirroring and the mirror stage, which has been elaborated in various ways by Lacan, Winnicott, and Kohut. Lacan appears to have been directly influenced by the new Hegelianism, through the lectures of Alexandre Kojève.[12] There is no evidence that Hegel directly influenced Winnicott and Kohut, however.

Second, Hegel described the basic asymmetry of intersubjective relations based on the inequality of desire. This inequality of need and desire leads inevitably to a fear of being controlled by the other, and eventually to a fear of psychic death at the hands of the other. Psychic death is equivalent to the loss of personhood: the self is submerged, swallowed up, or obliterated by the other. The relevance of Hegel's intuitions can be confirmed in nearly every contemporary psychoanalytic treatment. When I was investigating the experience of self and object in the so-called narcissistic personality, I described a focal dilemma in such cases that leads to a conflict between the wish to remain autonomous, self sufficient, and hidden and the wish to be known, to be found, and to surrender the self to the other. At that time I was unacquainted with Hegel and stated: "The psychology of the self is embedded in this fundamental dilemma, namely that the sense of self needs to be affirmed by the other, and yet a response from the other that is non-conforming or unempathic can lead at best to a sense of depletion or at worst to the shattering of the self. This results in a defensive quest for an illusory self-sufficiency which is in conflict with the opposite wish to surrender the self to the other, to merge, to become enslaved."[13]

Third, Hegel asserted that "the master is the consciousness that exists for itself."[14] This autonomy requires the externality of the other, which ultimately means the establishment of the foreignness of the other, leading to a wish for the other's symbolic extinction. Winnicott, in his paper "The Use of an Object and Relating through Identifications," also developed the idea that the autonomy of the self is secured only through the symbolic destruction of the other.[15] He added that it is necessary to have the assurance that both self and other have survived. Winnicott arrived at this perception through direct psychoanalytic experience, such as reaching the point of "maximum destructiveness."[16] French philosophers such as Sartre and Levinas, as well as Lacan, have adopted the convention of referring to the absolute externality of the other as the *Other*.

Finally, Hegel observed that the master who is omnipotent cannot acquire knowledge from others. Psychoanalysis confirms that those individuals who cannot relinquish belief in their omnipotence cannot learn from the analyst.[17]

The Multileveled Self

Until recently there were hardly any systematic, scientific observations of the newborn infant. Freud used the term "infantile" somewhat imprecisely to include all of childhood, and his description of the state of infancy, in the absence of scientific knowledge, was left to his intuition and imagination. He did think that infants are essentially self absorbed—that is, he viewed infancy as an autistic state. The infant and the mother form their own closed system that separates them from the external world. Freud, in a footnote to his "Two Principles of Mental Functioning,"[18] imagined that the infant is an example of a biological system totally under the influence of the pleasure principle without regard to the external world. He believed that the infant probably hallucinates the fulfillment of its inner needs and can ignore the reality principle because its mother supplies all of its needs. He analogized that this state is like that of a bird inside an egg, with its own food supply. In "Instincts and Their Vicissitudes," in accordance with his theory of primary narcissism, Freud stated that at the beginning of mental life the "ego is cathected with instincts and is to some extent capable of satisfying them on itself."[19] Self is differentiated from nonself by the contrast between internal and external stimuli:

> Let us imagine ourselves in the situation of an almost en-tirely helpless living organism, as yet unorientated in the world, which is receiving stimuli in its nervous substance. This organism will very soon be in a position to make a first distinction and a first orientation. On the one hand it will be aware of stimuli which can be avoided by muscu-lar action (flight); those it ascribes to an external world. On the other hand, it will also be aware of stimuli against which such action is of no avail and whose character of constant pressure persists in spite of it; those stimuli are the signs of an internal world, the evidence of instinctual needs. The perceptual substance of the living organism will thus have found in the efficacy of its muscular activ-ity a basis for distinguishing between an "outside" and an "inside."[20]

Following Freud, Margaret Mahler and her collabora-tors[21] believed that the newborn is in a state of "normal autism," a state of "primitive hallucinatory disorientation."[22] Mahler believed that by the second month of life the infant has a dim awareness of the mother and behaves and functions as though she and the mother were "an omnipotent system, a dual unity within one common boundary." Mahler therefore viewed early infancy as a state of undifferentiated fusion in which inside and outside have not yet become differentiated. This "normal" autism in the neonate is followed by a stage of symbiosis and gradual individuation. The process of individuation culminates in a sense of object constancy, which Mahler believed does not occur until the third or fourth year of life. Mahler implied that once the self is differentiated from the other, this differentiation is maintained as if it were a point of closure in psychic development.

Neurobiology and the young science of infant observation suggest a very different view of the infant's capacity to differentiate self and other. Edelman drew attention to the fact that there are two separate systems within the central nervous system, and that these differ radically in their evolutionary history. One is the system that can be said to form the neurological substrate for the experience of self. It is oriented internally and receives signals from areas that mediate homeostasis, whereas the structures that mediate the perception of the external world have a very different evolutionary history. This theory would predict that the neonate enters the world with a perceptual system that is ready to differentiate self from nonself. Observation of infants tends to confirm this prediction. Daniel Stern, in his overview of infant research, indicated that there is no substantiation for Mahler's description of an autistic phase and a symbiotic phase.[23] The infant is not enclosed in a common boundary with its mother. It can be observed to function as a separate entity that, in Stern's words, "exerts major control over the initiation, maintenance, termination and avoidance of social contact with the mother; in other words, infants regulate engagement."[24] Colwyn Trevarthen likewise observed that the infant can differentiate self from nonself almost immediately after birth.[25] There is no evidence of infantile autism. Instead, Trevarthen noted that the infant is actively curious in exploring its environment within minutes after birth. Furthermore, there appears to be an innate readiness to respond to the mother's affective signals. The infant is clearly "in the world" as a conscious participant with the mother, and not simply responding reflexively. There is, as Trevarthen described, a *mutual* comprehension of empathy.

The wish to merge and fuse with the other is usually interpreted as a yearning to recreate the blissful merger with the mother that all individuals presumably experienced as infants. It is possible that this wish for union may represent a kind of memory that is registered somatically at a stage of life the individual cannot recall. It is also reasonable to suppose that because the infant tends to imitate and mirror the mother's affects, and because the mother is attuned to the infant's affects, this synchrony of affects contributes to the illusion of a merging union.[26] This would mean that at some yet undetermined point of development, the infant has the capacity to experience the world at more than one level of reality: the infant can simultaneously experience both separateness and merging. With this capacity to experience self and other on more than one level of consciousness, such a self can be termed multileveled. Mahler's view—that the infant is originally merged with the mother and later experiences separateness—probably reverses the chronology. The experience of a merging union with the mother may *later* be superimposed on a perceptual system which all along maintains the demarcation of self and other. This split in consciousness may be a forerunner of the capacity to experience paradox.

A multileveled self is a self capable of experiencing illusion. Such a layering of consciousness can be inferred from the illusion of the transitional object, which is both a piece of objective reality and the infant's created reality. Winnicott said that illusions of this sort take place in what he called "potential space," a "resting place for the individual engaged in the perpetual human task of keeping inner and outer reality separate yet interrelated."[27] In the adult the capacity to feel at one with the other and yet be separate contributes to the paradox of being out of control and yet in control.

It may seem to be adultomorphic to attribute to the infant the sophistication of a multileveled self. But intelligent animals are also capable of recognizing multiple levels of reality. Gregory Bateson observed mammals in a zoo playing at fighting with each other.[28] He understood that this playing occurred within a frame that was demarcated from ordinary life—bracketed off from another level of reality. Animals have no problem recognizing that playing at fighting is different from actual fighting. If intelligent mammals are able to recognize other levels of reality, it is probable that this capacity is likewise present in the human infant at a protosymbolic level, before the acquisition of language.[29]

William James may have been the first to introduce the idea of the coexistence, in consciousness, of many levels of reality. He spoke of the many worlds of reality and illusion that coexist with one another. There is the world of physical sensation, the private reality of our senses; then there are innumerable shared realties: the reality of the subuniverse of science, the subuniverse of logic and mathematics. There is also a world that he called (after Francis Bacon) "idols of the tribe," our shared myths and illusions. Added to this is the supernatural world of religious belief, and finally the world of sheer madness.[30]

James also proposed that *"whatever excites and stimulates our interest is real."*[31] James's formulation suggests that there is a close link between interest and desire—that intensity of desire and intensity of interest bestow a measure of reality. It is in this sense that I believe Freud used the term *Besetzung* (cathexis) to indicate that libido was free-floating and could attach itself to nearly anything.[32] We speak of "passionate" interests, attesting to the fact that interests may represent a form of loving (see Chapter 5).

The Meaning and Function of Idealization

Freud believed, as did Plato, that we yearn to become part of those we love. Freud, however, approached the experience of merging with the beloved indirectly, through the topic of idealization. According to Freud, the ego (the self) is at first dominated by the pleasure principle; it takes into itself what it judges to be good and ejects what it judges to be bad. "Expressed in the language of the oldest—the oral—instinctual impulses, the judgment is: 'I should like to eat this' or 'I should like to spit it out'; and, put more generally: 'I should like to take this into myself and to keep that out.' That is to say: 'it shall be inside of me' or 'it shall be outside me.'"[33] Freud therefore believed that originally it is the self that is overestimated (idealized) and is the measure of all that is "good." The self, in ejecting what is bad, becomes according to Freud a "purified pleasure ego." In this way the self makes itself an object of love. "Thus the original 'reality ego,' which distinguished internal and external by means of sound objective criteria, changes into a purified 'pleasure-ego,' which places the characteristic of pleasure above all others. For the pleasure-ego the external world is divided into a part that is pleasurable, which it has incorporated into itself, and a remainder that is extraneous to it. It has separated off a part of its own self, which it projects into the external world and feels as hostile. *At the very beginning, it seems, the external world, objects, and what is hated are identical.*"[34]

Therefore, according to Freud, the self is originally an idealized self, whereas the nonself is experienced as foreign or alien and as such is hated. In this we can find an echo of Hegel's master/slave parable. Yet Freud's account of an idealized self that ejects what is bad and incorporates what is good can be true only for a very early stage of childhood. For older children not only identify with the "good" they perceive in others, but—especially in regard to their caretakers—also incorporate what is bad. The child who possesses enough discrimination to judge his parents' limitations as caretakers may need to preserve an illusion of the "goodness" of his parents by taking their "badness" into himself. Fairbairn noted this process when he said that the child would rather *be* bad than have bad objects.[35] Here idealization of the other serves several essential functions. By incorporating the object's "badness" into the self, the relation with the object is preserved. Furthermore, because the object's "badness" is brought into the internal world, the object is controlled.

This is one response to disillusionment; another response would be a withdrawal from the object and a substitution of the idealized self for the lost object. By incorporating the "badness" into oneself, one retains the object; by idealizing the self, one gives up the object.

Some researchers consider idealization a means by which the individual can cope with an ambivalently loved person by splitting the ambivalence into an idealized "good" aspect and a hated "bad" aspect. Melanie Klein viewed idealization in this way—as a flight from hatred, as the child's method of maintaining love for the hated object by splitting the object into good and bad portions.[36]

Freud asserted that love is hardly ever pure and unalloyed but is almost always mixed with hatred. He thought that the only instance of unambivalent love is a mother's love for her male child: "A mother is only brought unlimited satisfaction by her relation to a son; this is altogether the most perfect, the most free from ambivalence of all human relationships."[37]

Winnicott, on the other hand, claimed that Freud was idealizing the mother-son relationship.[38] He believed that the mother hates her baby before the baby hates the mother and before the baby can know that his mother hates him. In his paper "Hate in the Countertransference," Winnicott listed eighteen reasons mothers hate their offspring. In this context he recalled a popular nursery song, whose implications mothers fortunately do not grasp:

> Rock abye baby, on the tree top,
> When the wind blows, the cradle will rock,
> When the bough breaks, the cradle will fall,
> Down will come baby, cradle and all.

Besides needing to cope with the hatred of the loved object, the child idealizes the parent for the simple fact that it is only his caretaker who stands between him and a dangerous world. Here the leading motive for idealization is the child's physical helplessness.[39] To lose one's belief in the parent as a protective presence is to face catastrophic disillusionment. Children need to believe in parents' fundamental altruism—need to believe that parents will place the child's interests above their own. In many families, as we know, the child cannot count on this parental altruism; in such cases if the relation with the parent is to be maintained, it can be maintained only by virtue of denial and idealization.

In the best of families, there is an inevitable divergence of needs between child and parent. This conflict between the needs of the parents and those of their offspring is not limited to the human species. Recent ethological studies indicate that among birds and mammals, parents and offspring have widely divergent needs.[40] Altruism appears to have a genetic basis that is positively correlated with the degree of kinship. Altruism, therefore, is greatest between parents and offspring, but offspring share in only one-half of the parents' genetic material; furthermore, offspring are competing with the needs of current and yet unborn siblings. I have discussed this issue elsewhere with regard to the divergence of created realities between parent and child, realities that are constructed in accordance with this divergence of needs.[41] This limitation of parental altruism, to the extent that it is perceived by the child, is another powerful motive for the idealization of the parent. For idealization sustains denial, by means of which the tie to the caretaker is maintained.

In Freud's view, idealization, the overestimation of the loved one, is not only a means of preserving love but also a basic attribute of loving.[42] Freud traced the origins of idealization to primary narcissism, the primordial libidinal cathexes of the self. He suggested that it is the intensity of the libidinal cathexes of the self that is responsible for both the love and the overestimation of the self. This primordial condition is later modified, however, when the self and the ego ideal become differentiated.[43] The ego ideal then becomes the repository of this primordial narcissism. The self is no longer overestimated, but the ego ideal "is now the target of the self-love which was enjoyed in childhood by the actual ego. The subject's narcissism makes its appearance displaced on to this new ideal ego, which like the infantile ego, finds itself possessed of every perfection that is of value."[44]

Freud says, in effect, that one loves oneself to the extent that the self approaches the perfectibility of the ego ideal: love is contingent on perfectibility. But since the perfectibility of the self proves to be an impossible goal, individuals will seek to complete themselves by finding their ego ideal in the beloved other.

If we combine this account of idealization with that of the failure of idealization, which we call disillusionment, we can discern a circular or dialectical process. Children become disillusioned with themselves when their limitations become apparent, as the result of confrontations with objective reality. They then seek to restore self love by approximating the perfection of the ideal self. As adults, when this also proves to be impossible, they seek perfection in the other. When they become disillusioned with the other, they return to find sources of perfectibility within the private self, and the cycle of engagement and withdrawal repeats.

This oscillation between a union with an idealized other and a withdrawal into an idealized self has been confirmed in psychoanalytic practice. Michael Balint used this distinction to describe two contrasting character types, for which he unfortunately invented the terms "ocnophil" and "philobat."[45] The ocnophil has idealized the other and as a consequence clings to the object, whereas the philobat has idealized his own mental processes. Although these traits may form the basis for different character types, one more often observes a vacillation in the same individual between an idealized self and an idealized other. For example, a certain professional woman in psychoanalysis was at times extremely sure of her own judgments and did not hesitate to criticize the thinking of everyone in her field, including the most respected authorities. At other times, when in the presence of an idealized teacher, she was rendered nearly speechless and found it impossible to express her own thoughts, for she claimed that she did not possess any thoughts. She viewed this idealized teacher as a nearly omniscient authority who knew so much more than she did that she herself knew nothing; and (she felt) the little that she did know was worthless. She became disillusioned with herself and idealized the other, but this idealization led to a depletion of the self. At other times the process would be reversed: she would regain confidence in the superiority of her own judgment and would become disillusioned with and critical of her teacher.

Kohut ascribed this oscillation between the idealized other and the idealized self to a "bipolar" self in which there are swings between "a grandiose exhibitionistic self and an idealized parental imago."[46] Kohut's bipolar self is a self that seeks cohesiveness and completeness through a merger with an idealized omnipotent "selfobject";[47] but if that selfobject fails, whether through weakness or a refusal to permit a merger, the individual falls back upon a "grandiose exhibitionistic self." This selfobject transference, which self psychology claims is ubiquitous, is, as Kohut acknowledges, an idealizing transference. For, according to Kohut, the selfobject is the individual's experience of another person who assures the cohesiveness and unity of the self by being available as a source of "idealized strength and calmness."[48]

Psychotherapists and teachers are apt to be idealized, because their own needs are held in abeyance by the "rules of the game." Their primary role is to meet the needs of the subject.[49] The "rules of the game" exacerbate the asymmetry of desire that exists between therapist and patient. Idealization of the therapist is encouraged by the fact that for stated periods of time, the therapist suspends his or her own needs and devotes undivided attention to the patient. This is not true of any other relationship in ordinary life. The analyst, if idealized, may embody all of the virtues of the patient's ideal self, and the analysand may hope that by mere contiguity with the analyst, aspects of that perfection will be introduced into the self. This is rather like believing in magic—believing that contiguity with an idealized other will effect a transfer of those imagined qualities of perfection into the self. Most of us preserve some vestige of this belief, that through temporary identification with a powerful person we can acquire some of that person's "mana." It is not uncommon for analysands to believe that so long as they are in analysis, no harm will befall them. They have created the illusion of a magical connection with an all-powerful omniscient figure who will protect them from dangers such as disease, accident, and death. Elsewhere I have described how this belief in the analyst's protective power may assume a concrete quality, as if the analyst were a transitional object.[50] One of my patients, for example, who was approaching the end of a long analysis, insisted that I give him some small possession of mine, such as a paper clip, which he could carry with him as a talisman. This idealizing illusion may operate unconsciously; patients may become aware of it only when they are about to leave the analysis and are confronted with the fact that they are, existentially, truly alone and separate in the world.

Transcending the Dilemmas of the Master/Slave Relationship

I have used Hegel's account of the master/slave relation as an organizing principle in this discussion, because I have found that it is uncannily congruent with psychoanalytic observation and with research on infants. Hegel believed that self consciousness requires the consciousness of the other; and research on infants has shown that mirroring entails a matching of affect states, so that when similar affective states are shared, there is a physiological basis for the experience of merging. This constitutes one level of consciousness. As adults, we retain this capacity to share affective states, as can be seen in the contagiousness of affects. That is to say, in the affective sphere there is no boundary to the self. But those who are capable of experiencing the self as a multileveled consciousness will also retain the recognition of self and nonself; they will experience the paradox of being controlled by the other, while also being in control.

Merging and separateness can be seen as a dialectical process: with merging, there comes a counterreaction in which one reasserts one's individuality. The establishment of private space is essential for psychic survival, for one must avoid being swallowed up in the other. The therapist's empathy then becomes double edged; for if the therapist is always understanding, there is no place where, in Winnicott's words, one can remain "unfound." There comes a point in most analyses when the patient is unconsciously motivated not to communicate and not to provide the therapist with the clues that are necessary for empathy. I have interpreted this process as a form of symbolic actualization in which developmental conflicts concerning separation and individuation are symbolically recreated in current time.[51] At such points in the treatment, it may become essential for patients to establish the separateness of the analyst in order to reassert their own individuality. The principle here is that the reassertion of individuality is established through hatred. Freud said that the "purified pleasure ego" hates the nonself. And Winnicott claimed that "destruction plays its part in placing the object outside of the self."[52] Hatred seems to serve a complex function. For not only is individuation fostered by hatred of the other, but, in addition, hatred accompanies disillusionment. As Marion Milner said, hate is inherent in the fact that we do have to make a distinction between subject and object.[53]

In asymmetrical relationships, in which the other is idealized, individuality is threatened also by the fact that idealization of the other is accompanied by depletion of the self. What is valued is not in the self but in the other. The other is the person who *knows* and who *has*.

Belief in the other's altruism may have a paradoxical effect: if the other is selfless and without desire, the resulting asymmetry of desire strengthens the "masterhood" of the other and increases the fear of being controlled. The subject can of course escape this dilemma by seeking solitude and by simply withdrawing from the other person, or the other person may be treated as a nonintrusive presence who supports the subject's solitude. But solitude, a retreat into the illusion of self sufficiency, creates problems of a different sort, as we shall see in the next chapter. If a relationship with the other is maintained, then the question becomes: How does one relate to the other while preserving individuality?

This dilemma of maintaining individuality in public space was addressed by the French philosopher Emmanuel Levinas, who spoke of maintaining the continuity of the self in the presence of the other as a kind of indwelling, an "at home" *(chez soi)* where the self is not altered by the world.[54] The "at home" is a site where, "dependent on a reality that is other, I am, despite this dependence, free."[55] I take this to mean that "I am I" requires the integrity (and awareness) of the private self. To be "at home" with one's inner self is the opposite of dissociation and alienation. If one does not doubt the integrity and continuity of the private self, one is able to merge into the other, yet retain one's freedom. In this fashion, one can obtain knowledge from others without surrendering one's own private construction of reality.

In cases where the self is absolutely separated from the other, Levinas used the convention of describing the other as "Other." "But if the Other is the free one over whom I have no control, the Other is also a stranger who has no control over me. Freedom denotes the mode of remaining the same in the midst of the Other."[56] Levinas believed that *discourse* allows for the coexistence of freedom and union. Discourse is a "nonallergic" relation with otherness in which one can remain the same in the midst of the other. In discourse, the inner lives of both participants can be exposed and shared without any eventual decision as to submission or domination.

The Russian literary critic and philosopher Mikhail Bakhtin arrived at a similar conclusion.[57] He believed that the autonomy of the self in relation to the other is maintained in a "dialogical" relationship. Bakhtin included as "dialogue" not only speech but also the silent dialogue that a reader has with an author. It is possible to enter into the other through empathy, yet maintain "two nonfused autonomous consciousnesses."[58]

Winnicott's concept of "potential space" can likewise be viewed as a space that transcends the master/slave dilemma. If we include both participants, Winnicott's potential space becomes a space between mother and child in which play and illusion occur. It is a space that is neither the child's inner reality nor objective external reality. From the perspective of both participants, it is a space *that allows for the creation of shared realities*—shared realities that belong neither to the self nor to the other. It is a space in which mutually constructed realities are created. This presupposes the capacity to experience the self as multileveled.

In a larger sense, the master/slave relationship describes modes of loving, as well as modes of learning.[59] Both in loving and in learning, one may surrender the self to the other. But if one learns by surrendering the self to the other, one is not truly assimilating knowledge into the self but merely imitating the other. Aspects of one's private self must penetrate the knowledge acquired from the other, so that knowledge is translated into one's private language. It is only in this fashion that knowledge can become one's own. Freud saw that, ultimately, learning from the analyst is an act of love, that resistance can be overcome only by love for the analyst, that "the process of cure is accomplished in a relapse into love."[60] Freud therefore understood the confluence of learning and loving. This penetration of the self into the other and of the other into the self can be seen as a process of translation: the self translates the foreign language of the other into its own private language, or translates the foreign language of the unconscious. In a letter written by Freud to

Wilhelm Fliess on December 6, 1896, he described the various developmental levels of the mental apparatus as the place where *"a translation of the psychic material must take place."*[61] Psychopathology, then, would represent a failure of translation.

Summary

When we consider the self and the other as an intersubjective system, we need to examine two major attributes: the extension of the self into the other, and the asymmetry of self and other based on the inequality of need and desire. These considerations include symmetrical and asymmetrical relations between self and other, and the control and dehumanizing of the other that result from the inequality of need and desire. Merging with and idealizing the other are an expression of love, whereas the reestablishment of separateness may be an expression of hatred that is essential for preserving one's autonomy. Freud approached the subject of a loving merger with the other through the concept of idealization; indeed, he viewed overestimation of the other as the essence of love. Idealization and disillusionment can be thought of as a dialectical process. As a child, one becomes disillusioned with oneself when confronted with one's own objective limitations. One then seeks to restore self love by attempting to approximate the perfection of the ideal self. When this, too, proves impossible, one seeks perfection in the beloved other. When one is disillusioned with the other, one returns to seek perfection within the self, and the cycle repeats.

Contemporary neurobiology and research on infants suggest that, cognitively, the infant can differentiate self from other shortly after birth. Observations also indicate, however, that mother and infant unconsciously replicate within themselves the affective experience of the other. This provides a certain physiological basis for the experience of a merging union. I have proposed that consciousness is experienced at more than one level—that early in our development we learn to accept the coexistence of separateness and merging. This provides the basis for the acceptance of paradoxes, such as the paradoxical fact that we both maintain and lose control in our relations with others. Consciousness is multileveled with regard to the boundaries of self.

It is this multileveled self that provides a solution to the paradox posed by Hegel's parable of master and slave. The human dilemma implicit in the observation that one's assertion of individuality requires the negation of the other is resolved by means of a multileveled consciousness in which one is both merged and separate. While learning from the other, one can remain the same in the midst of the other, if one is able to translate the other's construction of reality into one's private language and thus preserve the integrity of the self.

5

Solitude, Passionate Interests, and the Generative Aspects of the Self

> I go and come with a strange liberty in nature, a part
> of herself.
>
> HENRY DAVID THOREAU, *Walden*

In the previous chapter we looked at self and other as an intersubjective ensemble. Let us now focus on a different aspect of the private self: the state of solitude in which one is sustained by passionate interests. Again, we are confronted with the paradox that although the coherence of the self can be sustained from within through the generation of passionate interests and moral commitments, the private self requires the presence of another.

The common definition of "solitude" is "the state of being alone." But the nature of solitude is complex, since one can be "alone" in the presence of another person. Solitude encompasses a variety of states that may range from pleasurable to exceedingly painful. In the latter case, it is termed "loneliness." Solitude (in contrast to loneliness) paradoxically implies that someone else is present.[1] Winnicott believed that initially the capacity for solitude requires the mother's presence: to be able to be alone as a child is an achievement. Winnicott proposed that the capacity to be alone represents a developmental step which requires a "sufficiency" of the mother's presence. Later, as adults, we are sustained in states of solitude by subjectively created (maternal) presences. In this chapter, I shall develop the notion that the muse is one such presence.

As Winnicott wrote, "The basis of the capacity to be alone is the experience of being alone in the presence of someone. In this way an infant with weak ego organization may be alone because of reliable ego support. Gradually the ego-supportive environment is introjected and built into the individual's personality, so that there comes about a capacity to actually be alone. Even so, theoretically, there is always someone present who is equated ultimately and unconsciously with the mother."[2]

Pleasurable solitude, then, implies that there is an internal contact with a protective or sustaining (maternal) presence—either an actual person or an imaginary one.[3] Solitude is a necessary part of our daily lives. For it is in states of solitude that we extend the domain of the personal over the impersonal. When alone, we are free to experience what is idiosyncratic in us. In this way, we reestablish contact with the private self and thus assure ourselves of the continuity of being.

The psychoanalytic literature regarding solitude is nearly nonexistent. Freud made only passing reference to the child's fear of solitude.[4] He discussed solitude in the context of objective anxiety, linking solitude to those phobias in which there is some element of real danger, such as a fear of traveling. Freud thus viewed solitude as a risk, but did not elaborate on the nature of the danger. He added that although solitude has its dangers, there are no conditions in which we are unable to tolerate it (though this ability may be only momentary). The dearth of psychoanalytic literature concerning solitude may be due to the fact that the experience of solitude is virtually ineffable. In solitude, we feel a stillness of the self that is very difficult to put into words. Susanne Langer, in *Mind: An Essay on Human Feeling,* suggested that this state is rendered less effectively in literature than in the visual arts. She wrote of "the calm, the spirit of eternal rest that comes to birth in an Egyptian statue or Mayan head," and described a Cambodian statue of Buddha as having the "living stillness" of a plant.[5]

Solitude is linked to the idea of privacy and to the acknowledgment that privacy is a human right. But privacy was one of the last inalienable rights to be recognized. This may have some connection with the fact that physical privacy in European households is of comparatively recent origin. As Philippe Ariès has demonstrated, physical privacy required that rooms be set aside as personal bedrooms, and this occurred only toward the end of the seventeenth century. Prior to that time, beds were placed anywhere in the house and no one was ever completely alone.[6]

Prior to the establishment of physical privacy, people achieved solitude and freedom from intrusion only when performing their religious devotions. In *The Varieties of Religious Experience,* William James provided many accounts of individuals who, in solitude, surrendered the self to the presence of God.[7] In fact, James defined religious experience as something experienced only in solitude—as "those feelings, acts and experiences of individual men *in their solitude* so far as they apprehend themselves to stand in relation to what ever they may consider the divine."[8]

If the capacity to be content when one is alone is a developmental achievement, it is by no means a permanent achievement. Everyone can expect to be overcome, at times, by intense loneliness. Loneliness can be defined as a failed state of solitude. But there is something puzzling about loneliness. It is not simply a frustrated yearning for human contact, since many people experience loneliness in the presence of others. Loneliness must involve some inability to experience a maternal presence. I once had a patient who was born blind and spent most of her life alone, but she felt lonely only when she was in the presence of people who would not make contact with her. She was quite content when alone in her apartment, surrounded by her familiar objects and her cats. But when she was away from home and her expectations of human contact were aroused and then frustrated, she felt intense loneliness. I believe that her cats and her familiar surroundings functioned as reassuring presences and provided her with a sense of the continuity of being.

Melanie Klein pointed out that there are individuals who experience intense loneliness even when they are among friends and are receiving love.[9] And we all know of people who have suffered great loneliness within marriage. Klein suggested that the experience of loneliness is an indication of unresolved paranoid and depressive anxieties. Conversely, she believed that loneliness can be mitigated by the internalization of a "good breast"—that is to say, a maternal presence.

Frieda Fromm-Reichmann was writing an essay on the subject of loneliness when she died unexpectedly, in 1957; the unfinished paper was published posthumously.[10] Fromm-Reichmann, who had an uncommon ability to make contact with severely ill schizophrenic patients, was impressed with the intensity of loneliness that schizophrenics experience. Some of her patients complained of loneliness so acute, so uncanny, and so uncommunicable, that they feared it as one might fear annihilation of the self. Fromm-Reichmann believed that this state should not be confused with depression or other forms of anxiety, but should be recognized as something in its own right. This intense form of loneliness, she believed, is underrecognized and underreported because it arouses anxiety in the therapist: therapists, too, dislike being confronted with their own loneliness. Fromm-Reichmann noted that, like solitude, loneliness rarely appears in the psychoanalytic literature. An exception is a paper by Gerald Adler and Dan Buie, who reported the frequency of the experience of painful aloneness in borderline patients.[11] They suggested that this sense of aloneness reflects the inability to evoke the memory of an affective object relationship. Again, this failure is similar to the failure to evoke an internalized presence.

Of course, in psychoanalysis one cannot observe absolute solitude. So that analysts' understanding of absolute solitude depends upon the reports of those who chose to be alone for extended periods—people such as explorers and naturalists. There are also accounts by those who did not choose solitude but who were forced into solitude through imprisonment. And there are people who have been locked within themselves by diseases that prevent communication; Oliver Sacks, in *Awakenings,* has described this condition in postencephalitic patients.[12] Those who seek solitude frequently report being replenished in this state. They feel something akin to the oceanic experience of being at one with the natural world. Anthony Storr, in his essay on solitude, cites the Antarctic explorer Admiral Richard Byrd, who sought solitude in order to "sink roots into some replenishing philosophy." Byrd related that when he was alone at a remote weather base in the Antarctic, he felt that he was at one with the imponderable forces of the cosmos, which are harmonious and soundless. "It was enough to catch that rhythm momentarily to be myself a part of it.

In that instant I could feel no doubt of man's oneness with the universe."[13] Thoreau, solitude's propagandist, relates in *Walden:* "This is a delicious evening, when the whole body is one sense, and imbibes delight through every pore. I go and come with a strange liberty in nature, a part of herself."[14] He took nature as his muse, and was sustained by his passionate interest in everything natural. He observed plants, trees, animals, geological formations—nothing escaped his attention.

When we turn to the accounts of those who have been forced into solitude, it appears that the resources of the private self have contributed to the survival of these individuals. What impresses us is their ability to sustain themselves from within in the absence of any human relationship. It seems that in extreme situations, some individuals are able to find sources of nourishment in the core of their being. A common theme of those who survive solitary confinement is that they are sustained by the coherence and integrity of their private self. Frieda Fromm-Reichmann cites the account of Christopher Burney, who survived, with his sanity intact, eighteen months of solitary confinement in a German prison during World War II.[15] "As long as my brain worked," he wrote, "solitude served a purpose." He was sustained not only by mental activity and rituals but by confidence in his political beliefs. *He was sustained by his passionate moral convictions.* His inner life became so complete a substitute for relationships, that when he was released he scarcely dared speak, for fear that people would think him mad. He created a coherent and predictable world in an unpredictable environment by adhering to a rigid daily routine of physical and mental activities. He manicured his fingernails, exercised by pacing in his cell and counting the paces, and forced his mind to work on intellectual and spiritual problems.

We know that solitude is essential for creativity. Although some creative individuals require another's presence in order to work, others need periods of nearly absolute solitude. Ludwig Wittgenstein is such an example. Ray Monk, in his recent biography, tells us that Wittgenstein found it necessary to isolate himself periodically from social intercourse.[16] Although Wittgenstein at times craved love and companionship, there seems to have been no one in Wittgenstein's earlier life whose presence was absolutely necessary for his creativity. He did have influential teachers—such as Bertrand Russell at Cambridge—who became mentors to him. But Monk shows that eventually a reversal occurred: the student outstripped the teacher, and Wittgenstein became Russell's master. At about this time (1913), Wittgenstein decided to leave Cambridge and live alone for two years in an isolated village on a fjord in Norway. He needed solitude.[17] Russell feared that Wittgenstein would go mad or commit suicide in his isolation. Instead, those two years proved to be among the most creative periods in his life—a period during which he *"had some thoughts that were entirely his own,"* as he himself said: "Then my mind was on fire!"[18] Isolation allowed him to have (in Hegel's words) "the consciousness of the master that exists for itself alone."

Wittgenstein's solitude in Norway was not absolute; he gradually learned to speak Norwegian and became friendly with some of the villagers. But, as Monk noted, he effectively removed himself from bourgeois society, from the obligations of ordinary social intercourse with which he could not cope. Most important, he avoided having to maintain relationships with his colleagues, *and thus he could have his own thoughts.* He was sustained by his work, by his passionate interest in understanding the fundamental—that is, the most primitive—principles of logic. There is also reason to believe that he was sustained by the peace and beauty of his surroundings: he took long solitary walks, which induced in him a kind of euphoria.[19]

With the outbreak of World War I, Wittgenstein enlisted in the Austrian army as an ordinary soldier. His motives for this step were undoubtedly complex. His sister Hermine believed that he wanted to take on some difficult and nonintellectual work—that he wished to turn himself into a different kind of person. I suggest that Wittgenstein was also seizing an opportunity to find solitude, to escape from his peers as he had done in Norway. This became a pattern that characterized the remainder of his life. In the army, Wittgenstein was separated from his social equals, but in the army one can never be alone. It appears that he created private space by distancing himself from his military companions. He did so by feeling utterly contemptuous of them, pronouncing them "a bunch of delinquents, unbelievably crude, stupid and malicious." He could scarcely see them as human beings.[20]

Wittgenstein was still sustained by his work, which occupied his mind no matter what was happening to him. Even while under fire, he preferred to be in a solitary and dangerous position rather than in the company of his comrades, for whom he felt nothing but hatred and disgust.[21] Although he was unable to continue writing his *Tractatus* at the front, he recorded his thoughts in a notebook and later used these notes for the *Tractatus.* Only when he was under direct fire did his philosophical musings cease. He complained that at such times he lost sight of his moral (inner) self and was, of necessity, overtaken by the animal instinct to survive, by the will to stay alive. When his tour of duty was over, he was assigned to noncombatant service for six months, during which he at last had an opportunity to arrange his notes into an actual draft of his book. Thus, in the midst of a war he was able to compose the *Tractatus!*

Wittgenstein was sustained not only by his philosophical work but also by Leo Tolstoy's *Gospel.* This book "kept him alive," since it allowed him to "leave his inner being undisturbed."[22] It assured him that whatever happened to him externally, nothing could happen to his innermost being.

Wittgenstein could tolerate the company of his colleagues for only limited periods of time, and periodically escaped either to a hut in Norway or to a cottage in Ireland. But as he grew older, he seemed less able to sustain himself entirely from within and increasingly needed the presence of others to keep himself from going mad. Friendships with both men and women had always been important to him; Monk describes several crucial friendships with male lovers as well as with women. His friend David Pinsent declared that "my presence brought him the peace which he needed while he was nurturing his ideas."[23]

Passionate Interests

Morris Eagle, in his essay "Interests as Object Relations," developed an idea that is similar to the one I am proposing and that Wittgenstein's extraordinary life clearly illustrates.[24] Eagle asked the question: What is it that sustains life? He concluded that in addition to love relationships, personal interests serve this essential function. Eagle further suggested that such interests permit the individual a measure of autonomy from the inputs of the immediate external environment, a view that is consistent with the functions of the private self described above. Research on infants has shown that individuals develop personal interests at the earliest stages of life. Infants and children, as they express their curiosity, routinely become fascinated with one particular object or activity in contrast to another. Such responses may be a result of their highly individualized nervous systems, which may lead them to become selectively interested in sounds, visual images, words, and so forth. Personal interests and preferences that develop at a very early age may later become the center of an individual's life. William James spoke of this center as a "hot place in a man's consciousness"; such interests can take the form of ideas or ideals, to which the individual is devoted and which become "the habitual centre of his personal energy."[25] If we combine this conception with Gerald Edelman's view of the brain as self generating, it follows that the individual creates his or her own interests. These interests can be thought of as emergent *values* of great intensity, which can become powerful motives in directing the individual's life. (This point is further elaborated in Chapter 8.) It is not too far-fetched to say that such passionately held interests are a form of loving. Iris Murdoch, in *The Sovereignty of Good,* suggested that efforts of attention directed toward individuals are an exercise in love.[26] The passion that some individuals invest in ideas, in moral values, in specified activities is analogous to a kind of love. There is something very useful in the idea of a free-floating libido that can attach itself to nearly anything. In this sense, a hyperinvestment of libido, expressed as a *Besetzung* (cathexis), is an expression of love. We could say that the private self generates private space through interests that claim attention and love.

Those who have a passionate investment in something outside the self appear to have a better chance of survival in extreme situations. Interests are something to live for; they make it possible to survive extremely punishing environments in which the solace afforded by human relationships is utterly lacking. Survivors of the Nazi Holocaust frequently claimed that what sustained them was a passionate commitment to some interest outside the self. The content of the interest was irrelevant. Adherents of Judaism, Christianity, Communism, and so on were all equally sustained by their beliefs.

Passionate commitment to something outside the self, such as a passionate moral commitment, contributes to the coherence of the self in times of great stress. For this reason, passionately held interests should not be confused with narcissism, although such interests may serve as a substitute for a loving relationship. Analysands may recognize this possibility, for occasionally patients will express the fear that to develop an intense interest might overwhelm them and enslave them, as a lover might.

Storr likewise emphasized the importance of personal interests that sustain one in states of solitude; his essay has helped draw attention to this relatively neglected topic.[27] But Storr, as a student of Jung, continued Jung's quarrel with Freud and took issue with Freud's presumed belief in pansexuality. Storr claimed that intense personal interests, if they are directed toward something inanimate, have nothing to do with love (taken in its broadest sense). On this point, I think he is clearly mistaken. Furthermore, according to Storr, Freud did not recognize the pleasure that such interests can bring to people's lives because Freud believed that heterosexual love was the *sine qua non* of human happiness.[28] Freud, however, was not particularly sanguine about the possibility of human happiness under any conditions.

Muses, Both Real and Imaginary

It is difficult to provide a precise definition of a "muse." Kohut's notion of the selfobject comes fairly close, since it emphasizes that the other person is there *only* to provide coherence and continuity to the self.[29] According to Kohut, a person will experience himself as a cohesive, harmonious unit in time if he senses other people as joyfully responding to him, "as available to him as sources of idealized strength and calmness, as being silently present but in essence like him, and, at any rate, being able to grasp his inner life more or less accurately so that their responses are attuned to his needs." The desire to see the other as a silent presence who intuitively grasps the private self, who knows *specifically* who you are, is derived from a wished-for maternal presence. The other functions only to affirm the self. This reflects an illusion concerning the other's total altruism, although it is undeniable that such altruism does exist. One must recognize that the relationship is a dialectic, including what the other brings to the muselike role and what the subject creates and attributes to the muse. As is apparent from many biographical accounts, the muse, when an actual person and not simply an imagined presence, is to a significant extent self created. The individuality and personhood of the other, the muse, are not relevant. The only function of a muse is to provide what is missing in the self; the muse contributes to the cohesiveness of the self.

Religious presences are also muselike, in that they are experienced entirely in accordance with the needs of the subject. William James said in *The Varieties of Religious Experi-*

ence that unless one believes in miracles, these presences must be considered "subconscious" (unconscious) creations.[30] As the title of his book indicates, James emphasized the *variety* of such experiences, giving numerous illustrations of the highly individualized nature of these religious presences. "The world can be handled according to many systems of ideas, and is so handled by different men. And why, after all, may not the world be so complex as to consist of many interpenetrating spheres of reality?"[31] James described a variety of religious conversions in which individuals felt themselves to be in the presence of a religious spirit described variously as God, the Son, the Holy Spirit, the Virgin Mary, and so forth. The experience might have been that of simply feeling the comfort of a protective presence; or the individual may have felt that his or her sense of self was given over to and swallowed up by the presence of the other. As a result of this merger with the holy presence, some experienced a sense of peace and harmony, whereas others reported that they had been cured of afflictions such as alcoholism and promiscuity.

James observed that in human consciousness there is a "sense of reality, a feeling of objective presence, a perception of what we may call something there."[32] It is this sense of presence that may have led the Greeks to ascribe to the abstract order of earth, sky, and sea the presence of a god who is the organizer of what appear to be coherent entities. It is the function of a god to bring order out of chaos. From there, it is a short step to believing that an analogous process occurs within the mind. *Chaos is organized by means of a godlike or goddesslike muse.*

Robert Graves, in *The White Goddess,* has provided the most extensive account of the mythical origin of goddesslike muses.[33] Graves believed that true poems have a "magical" quality, which he took as evidence that poets are possessed by a muse. What is magical is the ability of words to evoke a response in the body. True poetry evokes a primitive physiological response: one's hairs bristle and a shiver runs down the spine. Graves described a pattern in the poet's relation to the muse that is similar to that which James observed regarding religious presences. Poets may surrender and merge with their muse, or may stand apart. Graves believed that the true (Romantic) poet surrenders to the muse, the muse is his mistress "who commands his destiny," whereas the classical (Apollonian) poet claims to be the goddess' master.[34] Graves accordingly divides poets into "true" poets—who surrender to their muse, who surrender to the power of the White Goddess—and those who are masters of their muse. He is clearly contemptuous of the latter.

Graves believed that the muse was originally the Mother Goddess, who was worshiped before there were male gods and before there was even a concept of paternity. For in the earliest society, which was primitive, matriarchal, and polyandrous, no one knew the identity of his or her father. The White Goddess—originally a triple goddess, forerunner of the three original muses Meditation, Memory, and Song—was a personification of primitive woman, both a creator and a destroyer, both a black witch and a white witch. With the subsequent development of patriarchal societies, the original myth was correspondingly tamed, so that the muses were no longer identified with the primal mother goddess but were described as the nine daughters of Zeus, the offspring of a coupling between Zeus and the goddess of memory, Mnemosyne. These nine muses became obedient, and the power of the White Goddess became subject to the control of Apollo and his priests. Graves refers to these nine muses as "little departmental goddesses of inspiration," and sees this more recent myth as a civilized overlay that masks the primitive creative and destructive powers of the White Goddess. "A true poem is necessarily an invocation of the White Goddess, or Muse, the Mother of All Living, the ancient power of fright and lust—the female spider or the queen bee whose embrace is death."[35]

It is not surprising that this account of the White Goddess should correspond to Graves's own experience, for he is an example of someone who was completely taken over by his muse. Richard Graves, Robert Graves's nephew, has chronicled his uncle's fourteen-year relationship with his muse, Laura Riding.[36] She became in effect Graves's White Goddess, completely dominating and changing his life. An American poet of great intelligence, she demanded that those who were part of her inner circle unquestioningly and unhesitatingly accept all of her beliefs and values. She did, in fact, have a circle of admiring acolytes from whom she demanded absolute submission and control.

Robert Graves was initially attracted to Laura through her poetry. Without having met her, he invited her to join him, his wife, and their children as his secretary at a teaching post in Egypt. They soon became lovers, and eventually Graves left his family for her. He became her devotee, and completely accepted her constructions of reality. She criticized all of his work and altered his literary and personal values. He, in turn, believed that she taught him how to think clearly and how to speak the truth.[37] He worshiped her, abandoned himself to her. Graves idealized her for nearly fourteen years, despite the fact that at times she appeared to be mentally unbalanced. For example, she revealed to a friend that she considered herself to be "more than human, a goddess, a figure of destiny, she embodied 'Finality.'"[38] Some did accept her view of herself and believed that she possessed paranormal powers—that she was, in effect, a "witch." On one occasion she attempted suicide by drinking Lysol; when that had no immediate result, she leaped out a fourth-story window and nearly succeeded in ending her life. Yet due to his passive nature, Graves could not free himself of her until he found another lover. Even then, he did not completely break off his ties with her. Until the very end of the relationship, Graves continued to idealize her and to deny his hatred of her. His biographer suggests that this hatred was expressed in his poetry and in such creations as the malignant character of Livia, who, in *I Claudius,* poisons everyone who stands in the way of her ambitions.

Picasso was another great artist who had muselike relationships; but in contrast to Graves, Picasso stood apart from his muse. He would periodically free himself from his current muse and replace her with another. Biographer John Richardson has noted that Picasso completely changed his style of painting when he changed his wife or mistress.[39] The woman to whom he was currently attached appeared to dominate everything. Dora Maar (Picasso's companion from 1936 to 1945) said that when the woman in Picasso's life changed, virtually everything else changed as well. Picasso was intensely social and needed to be surrounded by a coterie of admirers, who were as vital to him as his daily bread. But his wife or mistress would determine who his courtiers would be, for they would have to be her friends as well. Not only did he change the composition of his court with a new wife or mistress; there would also be a new house, a new dog, new servants, and new food. Only certain essential functionaries, such as his secretary and his principal art dealer, would be exempted from this global transformation.

Picasso's style and intellectual convictions were also influenced by men, especially poets. A resident poet was always part of his entourage, for Picasso felt that constant contact with a poet would inspire him in his work. Guillaume Apollinaire, for example, exerted an immeasurable influence on Picasso's imagination and intellectual interests. Apollinaire was fascinated with harlequins, whom he saw as representing all of society's outcasts. Picasso shared this fascination, as well as Apollinaire's interest in black magic and sexual perversions. For fourteen years, until the time Apollinaire died, he was a source of solace and intellectual stimulation for Picasso. Indeed, Picasso's "rose period," in which he repeatedly painted harlequins and circus performers, could just as well, according to Richardson, be called the "Apollinaire period." It is clear that Picasso enjoyed the influence of a variety of muses of both sexes, but was not in thrall to any of them.

Richardson states that despite Picasso's dependence on his admirers, he was seldom able to relax outside his studio because a part of his mind was forever focused on his work. At times he would suddenly leave his friends without saying good-bye; he simply had to get away from people, and would lash out venomously if prevented from doing so. His friend Sabartes, however, claimed that Picasso never attacked him, "knowing that I understood his state of mind, and confident that I would not poke my nose into his inner conflicts; *each of us was a perfect example of solitude in companionship.*"[40]

Companionable Solitude and the Destruction of the Muse

What I am suggesting here is that the muse can contribute to the coherence of the self or, alternatively, that the self may be surrendered to an idealized muse. These polarities can also be observed in the psychoanalytic process: the patient may experience the analyst as a nonintrusive presence supporting the coherence of the self or, alternatively, may wish to surrender to an idealized analyst. More commonly, if the analyst is nonintrusive, he or she may function as a muselike presence, supporting the analysand in companionable solitude. In this phase of the analysis, the analyst is essentially created by the patient—is a subjectively created object.

In the initial stages of some analyses, especially in the case of so-called narcissistic personalities, analysands may present themselves as self sufficient and needing nothing from the analyst. Yet the analyst's presence is essential.[41] If the analyst remains nonintrusive, this state of self sufficiency can evolve into a state of companionable solitude. Patients may feel as if they are in their own cocoon, which is in turn enveloped by the analytic setting. I refer to this as a sphere within a sphere—a state of self holding within the larger sphere of the psychoanalytic setting.[42] The analysand is in a state of solitude in the presence of the analyst.

Classical psychoanalytic theory assumes that the limitation of the child's feeling of personal omnipotence comes about through a confrontation with reality. Winnicott suggested an additional explanation: he believed that the externality of the other, and with it the limitation of personal omnipotence, is linked to the destruction of the object. When the feeling of personal omnipotence has been limited, the child makes different use of the other. Recall the paradox implicit in Hegel's parable of the master/slave relation: that the omnipotent master, who exists only for himself, cannot make use of what he knows if he cannot learn from others. Winnicott believed that if the analyst is subjectively (omnipotently) created, the patient cannot learn from the analyst, because the patient does not recognize the other as a separate person.[43] Winnicott wrote: "In the sequence one can say that there is first object-relating, then in the end there is object-use; in between, however, is the most difficult thing, perhaps in human development; or the most irksome of all the early failures that come for mending. The thing that there is in between relating and use is the subject's placing of the object outside of the area of the subject's omnipotent control; that is, the subject's perception of the object as an external phenomenon, not as a projective entity, in fact recognition of it as an entity in its own right."[44]

One achieves separateness when one reaches what Winnicott called "the point of maximum destructiveness": "Study of this problem involves a statement of the positive value of destructiveness. The destructiveness, plus the object's survival of the destruction, places the object outside of the area of objects set up by the subject's mental mechanisms. In this way a world of shared reality is created which the subject can use and which can feed back other-than-me substance into the subject." This point of maximum destructiveness does not appear in all psychoanalyses; but when it does, it can lead to striking therapeutic changes.[45] Similar processes occur in relation to a muse. I have suggested elsewhere that the rejection of the muse may likewise serve to reestablish externality and individuality.[46] If the muse is banished, then one is again complete in oneself. When one reaches the point of maximum destructiveness within a therapeutic process, there is the reassurance that the relationship between patient and therapist will survive; when the muse is destroyed, however, the relationship may not survive. I believe that this need to destroy the muse accounts for Picasso's series of wives and mistresses. It is also illustrated in the following incidents from the lives of T. S. Eliot and Freud.

In his biography of T. S. Eliot,[47] Lyndall Gordon has shown that there were at least three women in Eliot's life who functioned as muses during his most creative periods. Eliot had a reportedly schizophrenic wife, Vivienne Haigh-Wood, to whom he was ambivalently attached; the guilt and suffering that this relationship generated were undoubtedly transmuted into his work. She was in a sense a negative presence, perhaps corresponding to the dark side of the White Goddess. In his essays, Eliot described "the horror that is projected from the poet's inner world of nightmare." He declared that his career was "a triumph; for hatred of life is an important phase—even a mystical experience—in life itself."[48]

Eliot's psychic survival depended upon the loving presence of an American woman, Emily Hale, who seems to have been his principal muse. According to Gordon, Emily was the source of Eliot's idealized nonsexual love: "Eliot was asking Emily Hale an extraordinary feat: that her feeling should match his own need to transmute love into 'Love,' a distilled concentrate that would never evaporate."[49] After Vivienne's death, Eliot nearly destroyed Emily by not marrying her, since she had had every reason to expect that he would. Eliot later found another muselike figure in Mary Trevelyan, who created a tranquil environment for him. But he rejected her as well and, in his sixties, unexpectedly married his secretary, Valerie Fletcher. In Gordon's opinion, the termination of Eliot's crucial relationships with the two (muselike) women, Emily Hale and Mary Trevelyan, may account for the decline in emotional vitality in his later lectures and plays. After his marriage to Valerie Fletcher, Eliot's creative life seemed to be over.

Freud's relationship with Wilhelm Fliess can also be construed as a muselike relationship that ended with total alienation. Peter Gay was puzzled by Freud's uncharacteristic credulity in his exchanges with Fliess.[50] For example, Freud accepted Fliess's almost mystical beliefs concerning the implications of certain numbers. Fliess believed in the existence of a twenty-three-day masculine cycle analogous to the twenty-eight-day feminine cycle. He further believed that the nose, a midline protuberance, was a dominant sexual organ that influenced all human health and sickness.[51] Freud readily admitted that in Fliess's presence he suspended his normal critical judgment. "You really spoil my critical faculties," he said to Fliess. This loss of critical judgment indicates, I believe, that Freud had surrendered himself to Fliess. He liked to say that Fliess's praise was "nectar and ambrosia."[52]

Fliess was someone to whom he could tell everything, and Gay suggests that Freud's need for Fliess may have been prompted by his lack of comparable understanding at home. Although Freud's household revolved about him, he felt very much alone; he could share nothing of his passionate interest in psychoanalysis with his wife, Martha. She was evidently a very competent and efficient *Hausfrau,* but, according to one of Freud's colleagues, she considered her husband's psychoanalytic ideas "a form of pornography."[53] Gay argues that Freud's wife made Fliess necessary. Freud shared his latest discoveries with Fliess. He discussed with him the most intimate details of his marriage (including the fact that he and Martha had stopped having sexual intercourse). Furthermore, he told Fliess of his anxieties concerning a possible cardiac condition—anxieties that he kept from his wife.

When the break-up with Fliess came, it was complete and permanent. In 1901 there was a final meeting, during which the two men quarreled violently. They never saw each other again. Freud later interpreted attachment to Fliess as evidence of his own latent homosexuality; correspondingly, he interpreted Fliess's reaction to the termination of their relationship as paranoiac. In this muselike relationship, when the point of maximum destructiveness was reached, the alliance died. Fliess became a stranger, an Other in the most complete sense.

Summary

One's capacity to sustain the self in states of solitude appears to be related to self-generated passionate interests and moral commitments. An individual may also be sustained in solitude by a muselike maternal presence, who may be an actual or imaginary person.

Passionate interests give people something to live for. Although such interests are self generated, they lie outside the self; in this sense, they are analogous to a loved object. Passionate interests can be thought of as emergent values, which can become powerful motivating forces throughout an individual's life.

The relationship between solitude and creativity can be seen in the life of the philosopher Ludwig Wittgenstein. Only in solitude could he generate thoughts that were entirely his own. Wittgenstein did not seem to need a muselike presence in order to sustain himself; not until late in his life did he come to depend on intimate friendship for the peace he needed while nurturing his ideas.

In other creative individuals, the generative aspect of the self may be facilitated by a muselike relationship. The function of a muse in providing for the coherence and continuity of the self is similar to the function of a selfobject as described by Kohut. The biographies of great artists such as Robert Graves and Picasso reveal two different patterns in the artist-muse relationship. Graves was completely taken over by his muse—he surrendered himself to her; Picasso, though he required muselike relationships, initiated and terminated them at will. Some creative individuals need to sever their relation to their muse in order to preserve their individuality and personhood; such a pattern can be discerned in the life of T. S. Eliot, as well as in Freud's relationship to Fliess. The privacy of the self is affirmed in states of nonrelatedness.

6

Process and Experience: The Unconscious Structure of the Self

> We eventually come to a point where the mental attributes we ascribe to a person will appear as states of the organism, or more specifically, states of its brain. When we do that, the person vanishes from view.
>
> BENJAMIN RUBINSTEIN, "On the Possibility of a Strictly Clinical Psychoanalytic Theory"

This chapter and the two that follow form a series in which I outline a theory of the *biological* agency of the self. As we have seen, Edelman's theory of the global functioning of the brain suggests a solution to the apparent paradox of the continuity of the structure of the self in the light of an ever-changing consciousness of self. Let us look now at the relation between unconscious memory structures and the creation of meaning. The vitality of the private self depends upon the capacity to generate meaning; the inability to generate meaning is a psychic catastrophe. I propose that the unconscious can be thought of as a neurophysiological process that has the potential to generate meaning.

From one point of view, the self serves the homeostatic organismic function of maintaining a continuous sense of identity over time no matter what happens to disrupt the integrity of the self. Yet from another perspective, the self is nearly coterminous with an ever-changing consciousness. The structural aspect of the self can be considered from a third-person perspective and thus can be the object of scientific description, whereas it is impossible to translate an individual's subjective experience into impersonal concepts without violating that experience. We have seen that Freud dealt with this problem by continually shifting from an impersonal third-person perspective (according to which psychic structures are neutralized energies) to an experiential perspective (according to which psychic structures are anthropomorphized as internalized persons). Fairbairn's theory of endopsychic structures extended Freud's anthropomorphic account, with important additions and modifications. Fairbairn theorized that the self is originally an organismic whole, a homeostatic entity, that subsequently splits as a result of trauma. Psychic structures represent the split-off internalization of traumatic *relationships*. Fairbairn in effect abandoned Freud's instinct theory, since he believed that impulses (psychic energies) are a part of and provide the dynamism of psychic structures. Impulses cannot be considered apart from objects. In Fairbairn's account the structures of the self memorialize "bad" object relationships, which include rejecting objects, persecuting objects, and sexually overstimulating objects. Both Freud's anthropomorphic account and Fairbairn's description of psychic structures as internalized object relations may be viewed as attempts to personalize psychic structures yet retain a scientific perspective. This anthropomorphism of internalized objects is, as we shall see, only a seeming anthropomorphism. Nevertheless, as Rorty observed, it is unsettling to consider an impersonal process that gives rise to the sense of personhood: "Psychological mechanisms look most disturbing and decentering when they stop looking like mechanisms and start looking like persons."[1]

But strictly speaking, psychic structures can never be personal; since they can never be experienced, they can only be said to *generate* experience. Psychoanalysis has identified a variety of psychic structures that correspond with specific functions: identifications, cognitive structures, affect structures, structures associated with defense, and so forth.[2] With regard to the unconscious structures that generate the experience of the self, it is difficult to think of such structures as anything other than specially selected memory systems.

Psychological functions can therefore be divided into experiential and nonexperiential realms. This division has been outlined very clearly by Joseph Sandler and Walter Joffe:

> The realm of subjective experience refers to the experience of the phenomenal content of wishes, impulses, memories, fantasies, sensations, percepts, feelings and the like. Implicit in this is the view that the individual may "know" his own experiential content outside consciousness; and that he does not know that he unconsciously "knows." All this makes necessary the conceptualization of the existence of what he can call a representational "field" or "screen" upon which content can appear to be assessed. It is part of the non-experiential realm to scan the material of the experiential realm *before it reaches consciousness.* In sharp contrast is the *non-experiential realm.* This is the realm of forces and energies, of mechanisms and apparatuses of organized structures, both biological and psychological, of sense organs and means of discharge. The non-experiential realm is intrinsically unknowable, except insofar as it can become known through the creation or occurrence of a phenomenal event in the realm of subjective experience. Affects can be regarded as falling within both realms, that which is experienced being the *feeling* component of the affect.[3]

Sandler and Joffe further state that "there is an intimate relation between the experiential and the non-experiential realms. The construction of a new percept, for example, involves the utilization of older structures and the creation of a new one. Thus new structures are constantly created."[4]

This notion of the way in which new psychic structures are created resembles the idea that memory is constantly updated by means of recategorization. Sandler and Joffe's model, in which psychic structures function outside consciousness to create a "representational field" that scans inputs, is similar to Edelman's model of the self, in which the salience of perceptual inputs is matched through the process of reentry. Further, their distinction between the experiential and nonexperiential attributes of affects clarifies the seemingly illogical idea that an affect can be unconscious—that an unconscious affect such as guilt can influence experience and behavior. It is fully evident that the unconscious realm of psychic structures, like categorical memory, contains *potential* for the creation of meaning.

Unconscious Structure and the Self

The idea of a divided self implicitly suggests that one portion of the self is unknown to another portion of the self. Thus, any theory of a divided self assumes that some aspects of the self are unconscious. Fairbairn's model contains a multiplicity of noncommunicating selves—the central ego, the internal saboteur, the rejecting object, the exciting object, and so forth.[5] The central ego and the internal objects replicate, within the self, earlier traumatic object relationships. These nonintegrated aspects of the self remain unconscious; the individual represses not isolated ideas, impulses, or affects but "intolerably bad internalized objects."[6] What is repressed is the entire gestalt of a relationship, recorded as a categorical memory.[7] Even though this internalized object relationship is unconscious, the thoughts and affects associated with this "bad" relationship have continuing potential to generate conscious experience. But the associative links to the original traumatic experiences may remain repressed.

This is illustrated by the phenomenon known as projective identification, observed originally in the treatment of patients suffering from severe disturbances of the self.[8] In this process, affects that are associated with the patient's past traumatic relationships are "placed" or projected onto the therapist, so that these affects are also experienced by the therapist. A split-off and unconscious aspect of the patient's self operates in a truly dissociative manner, frequently with the original traumatic roles reversed: the patient may enact the role of the aggressor, and the therapist that of the victim. But the fact that the patient's actions are dissociated makes it appear as if the affects that were originally a part of the patient's psychic reality were in some mysterious fashion "placed" within the mind of the therapist. Not surprisingly, there may be confusion in the minds of both participants as to whose reality is at issue.

In *Other Times, Other Realities,* I described an instance of projective identification. A patient of mine had a traumatic relationship with her father, who was given to unexpected, violent, and totally irrational rage reactions. When her father lost his temper, my patient, understandably, felt that she was the innocent victim, since she believed that her father's rage was totally unprovoked. It came, as I phrased it, totally out of the blue. My casual use of the words "out of the blue" triggered an episode of projective identification. During that particular session, I noted that the patient was very withdrawn and almost completely silent, yet she complained that I was not making any useful comments or interpretations. I replied, probably with a slight edge of irritation, that she wanted me to produce something "out of the blue." This comment of mine produced a violent rage reaction which I experienced as unprovoked, as coming "out of the blue." The fact that I felt I had made an innocuous remark which produced a violent reaction recreated in me the patient's experience with her father. I became the "innocent" victim. The patient believed that her relation with her father was "booby-trapped," because she never knew what she had done to set off the explosion. My patient perceived only that she was reacting to my irritation in response to her seemingly innocuous request. Only later did we learn she was completely unconscious of the fact that she was enraged and that she was acting in a very provocative manner. This aspect of herself was completely dissociated. Later, when my patient developed a more cohesive sense of self, she no longer generated projective identifications.

This clinical vignette supports Fairbairn's thesis that traumatic interactions are memorialized as a gestalt. It also illustrates the "scanning" function of the self, a process in which there is an attempt to match the salience of current experience with past categorical memories.[9] The trigger words "out of the blue" evoked, in the mind of my patient, a categorical memory of her father's temper tantrums. This categorical memory further led to the recreation in current time of a precisely orchestrated interaction in which certain connecting links were still under repression, so that from the patient's perspective an aspect of herself remained unconscious. This was not only a simple reversal of roles, for the patient also felt attacked by me: we *both* were attacker and attacked. Projective identifications show that affectively embedded memories can potentially be reactivated, a phenomenon that attests to the existence of unconscious affects.

There is an abundance of clinical evidence that indicates the existence of unconscious structures of the self. In Chapter 3, I described the decentering of the self, a state in which individuals become estranged from their affective core and feel that life is meaningless, empty, and futile. The fact that we speak of "decentering" rather than "dissociation" suggests that some different process is at work. This decentering of the self, this loss of contact with an authentic private self, can result from many and diverse causes. I have suggested that the defenses employed to protect the private self against intrusion from without may be turned inward and directed at the self. In closing oneself off from others, one may inadvertently close oneself off from oneself. This process is distinct from depression, although in severe depression there is an analogous disturbance of the self.[10] For in cases of psychomotor retardation, there is also an inability to generate meaning.[11]

This loss of contact with the deeper structures of the self can be observed in its most severe form in so-called borderline cases, where we may witness both a decentering of the self and a splitting of the self.[12] Winnicott observed that complete dissociation from this psychosomatic core of the self is experienced as psychic death.[13] Total dissociation from the deep structures of the self is an unparalleled psychic catastrophe, since one loses contact with the core of the self, which is the generator of meaning. If individuals are cut off from this deep structure, they are unable to attribute meaning to experience. Winnicott believed, for example, that in such cases attempts at suicide may represent an urge to actively recreate the *experience* of death in order to bring the earlier psychic death, a psychic absence, within the orbit of personal omnipotence—that is, within the orbit of meaning. "The original experience of primitive agony cannot get into the past tense unless the ego can first gather it into its present time experience and into omnipotent control now (assuming the auxiliary ego-supporting function of the mother [analyst]）．"[14] In such cases, physical death is seen as a lesser evil than psychic death. The phenomenon of psychic death is fortunately rare, but most of us, at least fleetingly, have experienced partial loss of contact with this deeper structure of the self, resulting in a sense of emptiness and futility.

Some borderline and schizophrenic patients describe persistent disengagement from the self as a "black hole." For defensive reasons, the self has compressed itself into nonexistence. As in the case of the astronomer's black hole, an implosion has occurred. James Grotstein has suggested that the term "black hole" signifies the patient's attempt to name the ineffable, to give a name to an absence that begets chaos, nothingness, and meaninglessness.[15] André Green earlier described a similar condition as a "blank psychosis," characterized by "blocking of thought processes and an inhibition in the functions of representation."[16]

A more familiar indication of the existence of an unconscious self is that of unconscious identifications. Freud characterized unconscious identifications in "Mourning and Melancholia," where he noted that the self accusations of the melancholic are not directed at the self but do fit someone else.[17] Such self accusations represent an unconscious identification with an abandoned object. When this misidentification is unconscious, individuals may behave as if they were the other person, and as a consequence they lose their own sense of personhood. It is a common observation in psychoanalysis that people's unconscious identification with a hated or rejected parent may exert considerable influence on conscious thought and behavior. Not only do such people behave like the parent but their behavior invokes in them an unaccountable self loathing.

The dynamic unconscious has been investigated using physiological methods.[18] But some cognitive scientists have insisted that it is a mistake to equate nonexperienced aspects of perception with the dynamic unconscious.[19] We do need to be reminded that all unconscious structures and processes are nonmental. We can define a structure as nonmental if it does not generate meaning. The following example of such a nonmental unconscious cognitive process admirably illustrates how complex behaviors can result from an unconscious neurophysiological process. Recent evidence shows that complex visual processes can occur outside consciousness. This phenomenon has been observed in individuals who have suffered extensive (postgeniculate) damage to the visual pathways, leading to a condition called "blindsight" in which the person is rendered phenomenally blind in one visual half-field.[20] Virtually all visual functions in the blind hemifield, however, are intact. If forced to grasp an object in the blind field, the individual will make preparatory adjustments in his or her fingers and hands geared to receiving that object—all the preparatory adjustments that would occur in a sighted person. There is evidence, then, that visual "perception" can be unconscious: such people do not "know" that they can see!

Christopher Bollas has introduced a concept that he calls the "unthought known."[21] Bollas has suggested that the memories of patterns of early mother-child interactions are laid down in the primordial self in a developmental period prior to the capacity for conscious recall. (Freud likewise believed that ideas could exist in the unconscious without their ever having been conscious. He termed this "primal repression.") Bollas is essentially offering a hypothesis about the origins of the embodied self, the unconscious psyche-soma. He suggests that this unconscious self is not without mental content that will influence adult behavior, even though such ideas may not be retrievable. The locus of the unthought known is Winnicott's true self, which includes the "mental representation of the mother's logic of intersubjectivity." Bollas proposes that the patterns of intersubjectivity between mother and child are internalized very early, before the acquisition of language and before there is a possibility of the recall of memory. The infant is imprinted, as it were, with the mother's theory of being and relating.

The Unconscious as a Neurophysiological Process

We know that Freud, when he was preparing his "Project for a Scientific Psychology," believed that mental processes and structures—such as the primary and secondary processes, the ego, affects, defenses, and so forth—could be described in neurophysiological language.[22] Whether or not Freud later completely disavowed this early effort to construct a neurophysiological psychology is the subject of a continuing debate.[23] We know that the "Project" was never published, and it is said that Freud attempted to destroy it. Evidently, he recognized that the primitive state of neuroscience at the end of the nineteenth century precluded the possibility of realizing his goal. According to a 1954 article by Ernst Kris, Freud decided not to directly utilize concepts taken from brain physiology but indicated that it would be possible to do so in the future; Freud believed that the terminology of psychoanalysis was provisional, valid only until it could be replaced by a physiological terminology.

Robert Solomon's reading of Freud has led him to the conviction that Freud remained committed to a neurophysiological model of the psychic apparatus: whenever he apparently abandoned his commitment to neurophysiology, this reflected the impossibility of correlating mental events with localized structures of the brain.[24] Solomon asserts that Freud abandoned not the neurological model but only the hope that *for the present* it would find neuroanatomical support.[25] Karl Pribram and Merton Gill likewise argue that Freud never abandoned these neurophysiological concepts; consequently, they claim, neurophysiology permeates metapsychological theory.[26]

Both Gill and George Klein asserted that Freud's metapsychology was so contaminated by neurophysiology that it should be totally discarded.[27] According to Gill, metapsychology is essentially neurophysiology masquerading as a psychology, and intention and meaning cannot be mixed with physiology; psychological propositions should be unadulterated.[28] Klein, in agreement with Gill, proposed that there were basically two Freudian theories: a clinical (psychological) theory, which should be retained, and a metapsychological theory, which should be discarded; for physiology and statements of purpose and meaning are mutually exclusive.[29]

On the basis of selected passages of Freud's work, it can be shown that Freud both disavowed neurophysiology and retained it.[30] For example, he insisted that his topographic model of the mind did not in any sense correspond to anatomical localizations. He also contended, however, that psychic energy was not a metaphor but a literal manifestation of a neurophysiological process.[31] Furthermore, the distinction between free and bound energy formed the basis for differentiating the (unconscious) primary process from the (conscious) secondary process, a distinction which Freud described as the "deepest insight into the nature of nervous energy."[32]

In considering the relationship between neurophysiology and psychoanalysis, Pribram saw this linkage as positive in that it would enable psychoanalysis to take its place as a natural science. Gill, on the other hand, felt that psychoanalysis should go its own way. Gill, like Klein, was convinced that it is not possible to include questions of intentionality and meaning within an objective science such as neurophysiology. There is, of course, a venerable philosophical tradition to support this position, as in the old distinction between *Naturwissenschaft* and *Geisteswissenschaft*—that is, between natural science and human "science."

Whether or not subjective mental states such as intentionality can be viewed scientifically has been a central controversy in contemporary philosophy.[33] Since I am not a philosopher, I am not competent to examine the broad dimensions of this question, which include the philosophy of language. Moreover, most philosophers of language examine public meaning, while the psychoanalyst observes private and personal meanings. So that "meaning" for the psychoanalyst is not quite the same subject as is the philosopher's "intentionality and meaning." This point will be discussed more extensively in the following chapter.

As we shall see, Edelman's theory of neuronal group selection, a theory of individual differences, suggests that it is possible to develop concepts regarding the psychobiology of private meaning. In addition, his model of the brain implies that objective science and subjective meaning are not separate domains. We may well be facing a radical reorientation regarding Dilthey's distinction between *Naturwissenschaft* and *Geisteswissenschaft*. If this reorientation occurs, the current debate regarding the "placement" of psychoanalysis—the question whether it is a hermeneutic discipline or a natural science—may be resolved. For there will be no inconsistency in a natural science whose field of observation is that of personal meaning.

It seems incontrovertible that if a process (or state) is unconscious, that process represents a state of the brain. Yet such a brain state has the potential to generate meaning—for example, in REM sleep. Freud's theory of the unconscious was also the theory of a somatic process (a state of the brain) that generated meaning.[34] In his paper "The Unconscious," Freud responded to an imaginary critic who asserts that only the state of consciousness could be described as mental—that the unconscious is a somatic rather than a psychological state.[35] Freud agreed that the unconscious could be viewed as a somatic state but claimed that it contains the *potential* to generate a mental process:

> We can go further and argue, in support of there being an unconscious psychical state, that at any given moment consciousness includes only a small content, so that the greater part of what we call conscious knowledge must in any case be for a considerable period of time in a state of *latency, that is to say, of being psychically unconscious. When all our latent memories* are taken into consideration it becomes totally incomprehensible how the existence of the unconscious can be denied. *But here we encounter the objection that these latent recollections can no longer be described as psychical, but that they correspond to residues of somatic processes from which what is psychical can once more arise.*[36]

Essentially, Freud proposed that meaning is in some unknown fashion *potentially* present in the unconscious as a *latent* property. The unconscious itself can be thought of as a somatic state from which the residues of memory can once more arise. As we noted earlier, Edelman's theory of categorical memory likewise posits that memory exists only as a potential.

Nearly seventy-five years after Freud, the philosopher John Searle arrived at a similar conclusion. In his paper "Consciousness, Unconsciousness and Intentionality," Searle argues that some but not all unconscious neurophysiological processes are mental. To be designated as mental, an unconscious state must be a possible candidate for consciousness and must have a certain "aspectual shape." Searle's use of the term "aspectual" indicates that when one defines subjective experience there are multiple aspects, multiple private meanings; for example, an individual's desire for water is different from a desire for H_2O, and this difference cannot be *exhaustively* known to an outside observer.[37] The term *exhaustively* is pertinent, for the private self can be known but not completely known to an outside observer. As Winnicott noted, there is an aspect of the self that remains unknown and unfound.

Searle maintains, as did Freud, that the unconscious is characterized by the *potential* to generate meaning. He therefore proposes a radical solution to the long-standing assumption that there is a fundamental divergence between *Naturwissenschaft* and *Geisteswissenschaft,* between science and meaning: "The ontology of unconscious mental states, at the time they are unconscious, can only consist in the existence of purely neurophysiological phenomena. At the time the states are totally unconscious there is simply nothing else going on except neurophysiological processes. But now we seem to have a contradiction: the ontology of unconscious intentionality is entirely describable in third person, objective neurophysiological terms, but all the same the states are irreducibly subjective. How can this be?" Searle answers this question as follows: "To the extent that unconscious states are genuinely *mental* they must in some sense preserve their aspectual shape even when unconscious, but the only sense that we can give to the notion that they preserve their aspectual shape when unconscious is that they are *possible* contents of consciousness."[38]

Edelman's Theory of the Self and the Neurophysiological Basis of Meaning

Searle's proposal that "unconscious states preserve their aspectual shape" is congruent with Edelman's theory of neuronal group selection, an evolutionary theory of the brain. Edelman argues that there is a distinct evolutionary advantage conferred upon those advanced organisms who have the capacity to differentiate self from nonself. Animals exhibiting *higher-order consciousness* have available to them memories of categorical matches between present and past experiences; thus, they have the capacity to differentiate the consciousness of internal cognitive processes from perceptual inputs arising from the environment—a capacity to differentiate the self from the environment. This differentiation is crucial because it frees the animal from the "tyranny of real time."[39] Edelman believes that primary consciousness is also present in human beings but is overlaid by the far richer higher-order consciousness of language, metaphor, and symbol formation. With the addition of language comes the ability to create a *coherent* internal model of past, present, and future.

Meaning enters neurophysiology as a biological concept through the idea of *value*. In Edelman's words: "Current perceptual events are recategorized in terms of past value-category matches. It is the *contrast* of the special linkage of value and past categories with currently arriving categories, and the *dominance* of the self-related special memory systems in this memorial linkage, that generate the self-referential aspect of consciousness."[40]

Edelman's concept of "value-category matches" enables us to understand how latent meaning can become manifest. As we noted above, Freud likewise believed that the unconscious embraces the "residues of a somatic process." Edelman's theory describes those "residues." His concept of value is very broad and perhaps overly inclusive, as it assumes a Darwinian continuum between humans and other animals. In humans, the possession of language explosively enlarges the range of value-category matches. For this reason, some might argue that the concept of value cannot be applied to those animals who possess higher-order consciousness but who do not have a verbal language.

Value is linked to categorical memories relating to appetitive, consummatory, and defensive behavior.[41] Memory is categorical and is recategorized through complex global current inputs, a process that Edelman terms "reentry." Since value is linked to categorical memories, value, as is true of evolution, is a "prediction of the past."[42] As Edelman observes, present perceptions, which are value free, become meaningful through a value-driven past. The very term "value," however, undergoes a change of meaning when the primary consciousness of other species evolves into the higher linguistic consciousness of human beings. With the advent of language, value-laden categories of memory become infinitely enriched. Categorical memories are overdetermined and make use of metaphor and metonymy. This can be seen in the associations to dream images. In his account of the dream of the Botanical Monograph in *The Inter-*

pretation of Dreams, Freud demonstrated how an expanding network of associations can be connected to a single dream image.[43] *An unconscious somatic process can be the generator of meaning.*

The capacity to recategorize memory, to modify the past in accordance with current perceptions, is linked to the unconscious structures of the self. When the self is dissociated or split, or when the self is decentered from its affective core, this process will be impaired. Edelman's newer theory of consciousness suggests, at the biological level, that meaning (the selection of what is salient in perception) is coordinated with the functions of the self.[44] Although we do not yet understand how neurophysiological processes are translated into psychological experiences, this theory of biological meaning is consistent with psychoanalysts' observations that loss of meaning accompanies the decentering and splitting of the self. In extreme cases, the person afflicted complains that all of life seems empty and meaningless. It appears in these instances as if the value-scanning function of the self has been impaired. Events in present time are given meaning through a retranscription which must extend to memories of the past.[45] If individuals have no access to affectively charged memories, they feel as if they are not psychically alive. In these disorders of the self, there is a failure of *Nachträglichkeit,* the retranscription of memories. In *Other Times, Other Realities,* I described the close correspondence between Edelman's theory of the retranscription of memory and Freud's theory of *Nachträglichkeit.* Freud's clearest exposition of this idea occurs in a letter to Fliess of December 6, 1896.[46]

One of the functions of the self is to reconfigure time, to juxtapose past and present experiences. Thus, according to

Freud's theory, the failure to translate memories from successive developmental periods results in psychopathology. I suggest, as well, that such a failure of translation (recategorization) results in a loss of meaning. I view the creation of "meaning," in the broadest sense, to be synonymous with what Winnicott called the "creative apperception of the world that more than anything else makes the individual feel that life is worth living."[47]

Retranscription and Representation

As I have tried to show in this chapter, it is difficult, if not impossible, to avoid the supposition that meaning is latently present in the unconscious as potential memories awaiting recategorization. A considerable body of clinical evidence supports the theory that the unconscious structures of the self can generate meaningful experience. It would be a mistake, however, to equate the *concept* of unconscious psychic structures with anything neurophysiological. There is a logical fallacy in thinking that a concept is equivalent to a process in the brain. Philosophers have coined the term "mentalism" to refer to this tendency to think of concepts as scientifically describable entities in the brain.[48] W. V. Quine says that if someone is thinking about Vienna, this thought is potentially describable as a neural event, but the general mentalistic predicate "thinking about Vienna" cannot be translated into neurophysiological terms.[49] I understand Quine to mean that if an individual is thinking about Vienna, this process could (potentially) be observed as a neural event, but that the grammatical construction "thinking about Vienna" is a mentalism and would not have a corresponding representation in the brain. Quine believes that mental events are physical, but that mentalistic language classifies them in ways incommensurable with the classifications expressible in physiological language.

Although mental structures are not equivalent to any physiological entity, we are entirely dependent upon such concepts. Without claiming any equivalence between psychological structures and neurophysiology, it should be possible to think about mental structures in a way that is commensurate with what is known about the functions of memory and to avoid such disembodied concepts.

For example, unconscious mental structures fall within the broad category of mental representations. David Beres and Edward Joseph define "unconscious mental representation" as "a postulated unconscious psychic organization capable of evocation in consciousness as symbol, fantasy, thought, affect or action."[50] But the concept of mental representation, as used in psychoanalysis, has a very mixed parentage and a very confused history, some of which can be traced to an antiquated eighteenth-century psychology. The term "self representation" has been used to refer to a fixed, static entity in the mind that *corresponds* to the individual's experience of self. This idea originated in the eighteenth century, in John Locke's view that atomistic entities in the mind correspond to objects of perception. A very different concept emerges if one thinks of a self representation not as a replication of perception but as a *generative* structure. The former idea is disembodied; the latter is not.

One of the achievements of Edelman's model of the self is his resolution of the paradox that defeated William James: the persistence of identity in the flux of consciousness. The continuity of the self is preserved by virtue of the self's linkage with the homeostatic brain systems: the self is the repository of a special value-laden memory system which, persisting over time, interacts with the environment, through reentrant signaling, in real time. Perceptions occurring in real time are recategorized through a "matching" with these value-laden memories. Thus, the memory structures that generate the sense of self must be continually updated.

John Hull's autobiography is a poignant account of how this process can be thwarted.[51] Hull, who became blind in mid-life, was nearly overwhelmed by his blindness but was able to recreate himself. He endured a prolonged period of mourning for his lost sight, often dreaming that he could see very clearly and having to confront his blindness anew upon awakening. He found it impossible to update his memories of himself: "I know what I looked like because of memories of photographs and [memories] of seeing myself in the mirror. So I know that my memories of myself are out-of-date and the strange thing is that I have no way of updating them. This means that I have a sense of cognitive dissonance when I think about myself. On the one hand, I know that I am such and such a person, with certain features. On the other hand, I know myself as someone who probably no longer looks like that, and I cannot witness the work of time upon my own face. How can I grow old together even with myself?"[52]

Summary

Psychic structures are by definition unconscious but generate experience; they contain *potential* for the creation of meaning. An abundance of clinical observation enables us to conclude that unconscious structures of the self exist. Furthermore, we can infer that these unconscious structures are organized around salient affective memories of interactions between individuals and their caretakers.

It is likely that the self employs a scanning function to determine the salience or meaning of current experience when matched with past categorical memories. If the self becomes decentered from its affective core, as occurs in severe cases of character pathology, experiences seem meaningless and empty. In extreme cases, the inability to attribute meaning to life's experiences becomes a form of psychic death.

I believe that it is both necessary and clarifying to think of the unconscious as a neurophysiological process. Current advances in neurobiology may make it possible, in the near future, to revive the goal that Freud attempted to realize in his "Project for a Scientific Psychology": to describe psychological events in the language of neurophysiology. In his paper "The Unconscious," Freud acknowledged that the unconscious represents a somatic process, but a process in which latent meaning is embedded. A similar view has recently been proposed by John Searle, who also believes that unconscious mental states are purely neurophysiological phenomena. Unconscious states that are mental can be distinguished from unconscious states that are nonmental by their *latent* capacity to generate meaning.

As a result of this convergence of recent knowledge gained from neurophysiology, philosophy, and psychoanalysis, we are beginning to assemble the elements that may eventually lead to a biology of meaning. A biology of meaning can be derived from Edelman's concept of value. Edelman defines "value" as evolutionary constraints favoring behavior that fulfills homeostatic requirements or increases fitness. Value is linked to categorical memories relating to appetitive, consummatory, and defensive behavior. Current perceptual events are recategorized in terms of past value-category matches. The self, through this matching and scanning process, assigns value to current experience.

One must be careful to avoid equating unconscious psychic structures with neurophysiological entities. Nevertheless, it is now possible to think about mental structures in a way that is commensurate with neurophysiological knowledge about the nature of memory. Freud's concept of *Nachträglichkeit* and Edelman's theory of memory as recategorization suggest that unconscious structures of the mind must be considered generative and not static.

7

Private Meaning and the Agency of the Self

Where It is I shall be.
> SIGMUND FREUD, "New Introductory Lectures on Psychoanalysis"

The original experience of primitive agony cannot get into the past tense unless the ego can first gather it into its own present time experience.
> DONALD W. WINNICOTT, *Psychoanalytic Explorations*

Let us now look at the relation between the personal and impersonal, with special reference to the role of affects and memory. In this chapter I shall link affects, meaning, and the agency of the self. The concept of biological value will enable us to move effortlessly from value as an evolutionary property to meaning in a psychological context.

The term "agency" suggests effectiveness—suggests that one is not coerced by impersonal forces and that one has the option of living one's life. The epigraphs to this chapter point to the instrumentality of the self. Both refer to an aim of psychoanalysis: to extend the agency of the self through the creation of meaning.

I define "meaning" here as "personal significance." (There are, of course, many other ways of defining it.)[1] In psychoanalytic treatment, the agency of the self is extended when *new meanings are created*—or, to put it differently, *when old memo-*

ries are recategorized. This recategorization of old memories is facilitated by means of the psychoanalytic setting and the patient's new relationship with the analyst.[2]

Meaning in psychoanalysis always refers to what is significant for the analysand. Even when meanings are arrived at through shared (public) experiences with the analyst, they are always referred back to the analysand. What gives an item significance (for both participants) in a psychoanalytic treatment is the extent to which speech or other forms of behavior are invested with feeling. The analyst listens to the patient's speech and observes the totality of the patient's behavior, including posture, bodily movements, and silences. From these items an affective charge is communicated that directs the analyst's attention and interest to what is meaningful to the patient. We customarily think of the analyst's empathy as analogous to a perceptual instrument, but in order to activate this instrument a certain quantum of affective charge is required. (I have discussed this topic in *Psychoanalysis in a New Context.*)[3] If the patient does not communicate feeling in speech, gestures, or other forms of behavior, the analyst is unable to enter into the patient's experience. Without the affective inflections of speech, all words become of equal significance and are shorn of their personal meaning.

It is clear, then, that within the context of psychoanalysis the term "meaning" is equivalent to personal (private) meaning. Theories of meaning have been within the domain of philosophy for two thousand years. According to the traditional view, there is a rational structure of the world independent of individual beliefs—that is, independent of privately generated meanings. Many linguists and philosophers of language believe that meaning is not private, personal, or experiential. If meaning is considered as existing apart from feeling and desire, it is disembodied.

The linguist George Lakoff, in *Women, Fire, and Dangerous Things,* and the philosopher Mark Johnson, in *The Body in the Mind,* have challenged this traditional view of meaning, which they refer to as a "God's-Eye View."[4] In this "objectivist" or "God's-Eye View," words are signs or arbitrary symbols, meaningless in themselves but acquiring meaning from their capacity to correspond to things in the world. In other words, in traditional accounts meaning has been defined as impersonal and public. Johnson has argued that without imagination, nothing in the world could be meaningful; without imagination, we can never make sense of experience. Both authors emphasize that metaphors derived from the kinesthetic experience of the self-schema of our bodies give meaning to speech and language. For example, the meaning of "in and out" is derived from the kinesthetic experience of our body as a container demarcating the self from the nonself. Lakoff has described how the feeling of anger creates verbal metaphors that reflect the kinesthesia of the bodily experiences of anger.[5] Anger is experienced as heat, pressure, the need for containment, and so forth. These bodily experiences generate myriad structurally related expressions denoting anger. The work of Lakoff and Johnson adds to the evidence showing that *metaphor is the currency of the mind.*[6]

Another philosopher of language who views meaning as inseparable from biology is Ruth Millikan. She views language as a "normal" function, a product of evolution; for inanimate objects cannot be described as "normal" or "abnormal." In *Language, Thought, and Other Biological Categories,* she considers the relation between private and public meaning.[7] Private meaning is a kind of translation from public meaning. Millikan states that when a speaker takes over a public-language term, he must develop an inner program that matches the public function of that term. He must learn to translate the outer term into an inner term that has the same sense as the outer, and vice versa.

The Norwegian psychologist Ragnar Rommetveit has likewise considered the relation between personal meaning and public meaning.[8] Since every person has the capacity to develop an individualized perspective, meaning is created within the private domain of experience. In this sense, everyone inhabits many possible worlds. As Rommetveit says, "The problem *of what is being meant by what* is said cannot any longer be pursued in terms of stipulated unequivocal 'literal' meanings. The basic riddle is rather how states of intersubjectivity and shared social reality can be attained in encounters between different 'private worlds.'"[9]

The relation between private worlds and intersubjectivity is one that the psychoanalyst is particularly well positioned to observe. As we have seen, there are patients whose survival depends on preserving their own construction of reality, preserving their own world of private meaning in opposition to the intrusion of alien constructions of reality. This includes, of course, the analyst's construction of reality.[10] We shall return to this topic below.

Lakoff and Johnson suggest that a language contains certain metaphors that are in the public domain because they are derived from shared and nearly universal kinesthetic experiences of the body. A theory that locates the origin of meaning in personal experience, in the kinesthetic experience of the body, is similar to the psychoanalytic conception that meaning is linked to affective experience. Whether meaningful affective experiences contribute to the coherence or agency of the self will depend on the degree to which they are recategorized. For example, a patient of mine had been repeatedly beaten by her abusive father when she was a child. Subsequently, in her relations with men, this woman always anticipated a potential for abuse or humiliation. No matter what the experience was, she was compelled to scan every encounter with a man in order to focus upon those items that were potentially damaging, destructive, or humiliating. She compulsively examined current perceptions for a categorical match with her abusive relationship with her father. Novelty was disturbing to her and was apt to be minimized or dismissed. As is common in cases of trauma, she foreshortened and telescoped current perceptions into the past, and her past determined future expectations. She was in thrall to old memories and to old meanings. In this instance, the self was constricted because trauma impaired the capacity to create new meanings.

I believe that *the coherence and continuity of the self are augmented when the self extends its agency through the creation of new meaning.* The individual creates new meanings through experiencing the cyclical nature of time: the present transforms the past, and the past informs the present.[11] As a result of trauma, under the dominating influence of those memories there may be a constriction of the self's agency and a resultant constriction in the creation of new meaning.

I suggested in *Other Times, Other Realities* that the compulsion to repeat is a function not of instinct, as Freud believed, but of memory. An individual will continue to compulsively scan perceptions for categorical matches with past traumatic experiences until such memories are recategorized. In accordance with Edelman's theory of categorical memory, I described my patient's anticipation of abuse as an "affect category."[12] In cases of trauma, affect categories are compulsively imposed on current perception; current perceptions are then shoehorned into these old affect categories so that differences between past and present become minimal. There is a bias against novel perceptions.

Whether affective experiences support or diminish the agency of the self is a topic that Freud frequently explored using a different language—the language of the ego rather than of the self. Freud implied the existence of agency when he referred to the "taming" of the instincts by the ego. Psychoanalytic research, he said, proved that "the ego is not even master in its own house, but must content itself with scanty information of what is going on unconsciously in its mind."[13] Freud saw this affront to the human being's narcissism as one of a series of blows inflicted by science. Copernicus and Darwin destroyed the belief that humans are at the center of the universe, and psychoanalysis destroyed the belief that one is the master of one's own soul. As Richard Rorty has said, this decentering indicates what is most unsettling about psychoanalysis: Freud suggested not only that one is not master of one's own house but that one's house is occupied by alien presences.[14]

"Where It Is I Shall Be"

When Freud wrote "Where It is I shall be,"[15] he was using "It" in the sense formulated by Georg Groddeck, who introduced the term. "It" is the impersonal, attesting to the fact that we are "lived" by unconscious and uncontrollable forces.[16] Freud portrayed this It (id) as "a chaos, a cauldron full of seething excitations."[17] He emphasized that the major threat to the ego's continuity and coherence was internal. Today most psychoanalysts would give equal weight to the threats from without—to developmental disturbances and traumatic impingements, all of which result in a loss of a sense of the agency of the self. This loss of the sense of agency reflects a decline in the self's coherence. "Coherence" literally means "a sticking together," so that a severe disturbance of homeostasis implies a fragmentation of the self, a flying apart, a sense of chaos. When Freud spoke of the irrational and chaotic id, he believed that the ego gained mastery over the id developmentally through a process of internalization. Freud referred to this process as a "desexualization" or "sublimation" where, through identification, the ego assumes the features of the loved object and forces itself upon the id, saying: "Look, you can love me, too—I am so like the object."[18] In current time, in contrast to early development, the I (ego) extends its hegemony over the It (id) by means of insight. In psychoanalytic treatment, insight is achieved both by means of those interpretations that make the unconscious conscious and by a reliving within the transference. All of these measures extend the agency of the self.

Clinical observations suggest that when affects are experienced as outside the agency of the self, they are felt to be a danger to the self. Such affects may be without mental content, unspecified and unnamed. Contentless affects are liable to be experienced somatically. For example, anxiety may not be recognized as such when it appears as diarrhea, nausea, or severe muscle tension. The somatic expression of affects may be outside the agency of the self, and such affective experiences tend to be intrusive. But if affects are named and have an ideational content, if anger, guilt, anxiety, and sexual desire are accompanied by specific thoughts and fantasies, those affects are imbued with personal significance. Furthermore, some individuals believe that specific affects are within the domain of the self whereas other affects are not. For example, a patient of mine explained that if one becomes angry this can be controlled, but experiencing love renders one helpless.

Naming and uncovering mental content facilitate the sense of agency. For this reason, psychoanalytic therapists consistently attempt to uncover the mental content of affective experiences. Some patients require that the analyst identify—that is, name—their affects. Patients may be aware only of somatic sensations or of a generalized and vague sense of arousal and discomfort; they may be unable to name what they are feeling. Therapists, by means of their countertransference, can identify affects that are unconsciously communicated by the patient. In such cases it is the psychoanalyst who names what the patient is feeling: "You are angry," "You are feeling anxious," "You are sad," and so forth. The therapist is in effect teaching patients to name their own affects and thereby bring those affects within the domain of the self. I have described this process in *Other Times, Other Realities.*[19]

In some cases it is possible to attribute this inability to name affective experiences to a missing element in the patient's relationship with the mother. It is reasonable to suppose that the unconscious mirroring of the child's affective response by the mother, a phenomenon that has been widely reported by researchers on infants, is missing in these cases.[20] Such patients report that their mothers appear to be unaware of what their children are feeling and consequently cannot assist them in naming their affects. When the mother unconsciously replicates the infant's affective state, this replication may serve a protolinguistic naming function. The imitation of the baby's affects precedes as well as accompanies the mother's imitating the baby's speech as "baby talk." Lakoff has noted that the Tahitians do not have a word for sadness and consequently have no way of coping with sadness and depression.[21] They attribute sadness to something outside the self and categorize it with sickness, fatigue, and attacks by evil spirits.

The homeostasis of the self is disturbed not only by unassimilated affects but also by unassimilated experiences that we label traumatic. In "Beyond the Pleasure Principle" Freud offered, in his account of a child's game, a paradigm of the mastery of trauma through the individual's ability to create a symbolic model of the traumatic interaction.[22] Freud's theory encompasses what Winnicott would later call "gathering impingements into the area of omnipotence."[23] Freud's description of the child's game supports the thesis that it is through the creation of private meaning that one extends the domain of the self. It should be noted, parenthetically, that Freud did not claim the child's game created new meanings. Instead, he interpreted the child's game as a demonstration that the need for active mastery takes precedence over the pursuit of pleasure.

The trauma that Freud depicted is that of the child's separation from its mother. Freud was living under the same roof with a one-and-a-half-year-old child, his grandson.[24] This child was greatly attached to his mother, who, on occasion, would leave him. Her departure was followed by a game in which the child would throw a wooden reel over the edge of his cot so that it disappeared into it; at the same time he would utter, "O-o-o-o." Freud surmised that this exclamation was not meaningless baby talk but was the child's version of the German word *fort* ("gone"). The child would then pull the reel out of the cot with the joyful exclamation *"Da!"* ("There!"). Freud interpreted this game as the child's great "cultural achievement," a triumph over the instinctual wish to possess his mother completely and prevent her departure. By staging this game, the child symbolically controlled the mother's departure and return, removing the trauma of his mother's absence into the "omnipotence" of the self.

Also of special interest is that the game illustrated a transitional stage between a private "language" and public language. This child did not utter the word *fort* but instead said "O-o-o-o," which stood for *fort* but was the child's own creation. The child's game, then, consisted of a mixture of private symbolic gestures and public language.[25]

Meaning and the Recategorization of Trauma

In the previous chapter, I referred to the essay "Fear of Breakdown," in which Winnicott discussed what one might call the failure of recategorization. Winnicott described a patient who sought suicide as an adult, apparently as a consequence of a disintegration of the self experienced in childhood. The patient could not bring this overwhelming trauma within the agency of the self and felt it as a psychic death. In Winnicott's view, the patient's wish to commit suicide was an effort to master a passively experienced psychic death by actively bringing about an actual death: "The original experience of primitive agony cannot get into the past tense *unless the ego can first gather it into its own present time experience.*"[26] This inability to recategorize the traumatic experience was in effect an inability of the self to create new meaning, a failure that resulted in a massive sense of futility and emptiness.

As we have seen, there are two characteristic pathologies of the self that can disrupt its homeostasis: splitting and de-centering. Both conditions can be viewed as a deformation of the self in the service of defense. Traumatic interactions with caretakers are internalized so that the self may become its own persecutor. To preserve the cohesion of the self, these alien aspects of the self are repressed. When repression is massive and extensive, the recategorization of affective memories will be impeded, and this interference will in turn block entire areas of private meaning. If one's life is dominated by a self in which some other person is behaving as if he or she is in charge, the self has obviously lost its sense of agency.[27] These "alien presences" within the self, to the extent that they interfere with the coherence of the self, result in a *constriction of private meaning*.

In the decentering of the self, the generation of private meaning is disturbed in a somewhat different fashion. The private self has an affective core which needs to be protected from unempathic intrusions. This "protector" self is the same as Winnicott's "false self." Here, the means used to protect the private self from intrusion by others—a certain falseness, inauthenticity, and noncommunication of affects—are recreated within the self. One becomes estranged from one's affective core and is as false and inauthentic within oneself as one is with others. In the struggle to preserve private space, one achieves a tragic pyrrhic victory. Private meanings cannot be generated, since the self is out of touch with affective valences. If this process becomes extensive, one feels empty, lacking any defining interests or personal values. Life itself has no meaning.

In healthy individuals there appears to be a circular, self-reinforcing, synergic process between the self as a whole and affective centering. The affective centering of the self enables it to bring experience within its domain; to the extent that this is possible, the center is reinforced. If the center is reinforced, meaning can be further extended.

What has meaning for us has interest and hence is of value. Edelman defines "value" as those evolutionary constraints favoring behavior that fulfills the requirements of homeostasis or increases fitness.[28] Affects are the internal value-laden signals that ensure survival. Evolutionary values therefore inform conscious experience by means of affects. Such affects include not only pleasure and pain but also specific unlearned anxieties that provide the individual with an adaptive advantage. In the human species and other primates, for example, separation anxiety is such a genetically determined affect signal. Edelman's theory of value and reentry, and Freud's theory of affects, are both essentially historical concepts. Freud believed that affects are historical markers both in evolutionary time and in the history of the individual.[29] Edelman's theory of value likewise encompasses somatic and evolutionary time. Since values are both given and self generating, the concept of value includes ever-increasing levels of complexity—from the level of biology, to the psychological level, and finally to the level of culture and society. *If one accepts the hypothesis that affects are internal value-laden signals essential for survival, there is a clear progression from value as an evolutionary property to affects and meaning in the psychological domain.*

Private Meaning and Divergent Constructions of Reality

In private space the self is fueled from within through creative apperception, passionate interests, and moral values. In the context of this chapter, we can say that the self replenishes itself through the creation of meaning. For this to occur, the area of private space must be safeguarded from intrusion. The personal construction of reality contributes to the sense of being psychically alive. In some cases the preservation of this private construction of reality is essential for psychic survival—especially so if the child has caretakers who have an unreliable construction of reality or are excessively intrusive.[30] That the preservation of private space and personal meaning is essential for survival can be observed most clearly in cases of trauma or child abuse. It has been noted that children can withstand trauma more successfully if they have the ability to fantasize.[31] In such cases children retain the capacity to translate traumatic experiences into their own private thoughts (as in the game played by Freud's grandson) and thus bring the trauma within the control of the self.

The inability to translate traumatic experiences into one's private "language" is a subject that was originally investigated by Sándor Ferenczi in connection with the sexual abuse of children by adults.[32] In his paper "Confusion of Tongues between Adults and the Child," Ferenczi discussed the child's confusion resulting from the contrast between his or her "language of tenderness" and the adult's language of "passion, lust, and hypocrisy." The child's inability to translate the adult's conception of reality is more widespread than Ferenczi assumed; it is not limited to cases of sexual seduction or other forms of abuse.[33] The divergent constructions of reality in the adult and the child are due not only to differences in maturity but also to the unavoidable fact that parent and child have different needs. Parental altruism, the suspension of one's needs in favor of the child's needs, is at best only relative. This view receives support from a branch of evolutionary biology known as "kinship theory."

Some children become aware of this divergence of need and perceive that their parent's construction of the world may not be in their own interests—an awareness that is most likely to develop when one or both parents are severely disturbed or mentally ill. In such cases, children can survive psychically only by retaining their own construction of reality; their capacity to preserve themselves through the creation of a world of private meanings is life sustaining. Such children need to remain within their own "secret garden."

They pay a price, however, if in order to preserve private meaning they lose the ability to translate other constructions of reality. In psychoanalysis, one does encounter individuals who have been so traumatized that they cannot take in anything from others that they have not already thought of themselves.[34] If in order to preserve the coherence of the self one must exclude other versions of reality, one's ability to learn from others will be impaired.

Multiple Levels of Consciousness and Degrees of Freedom

New meanings are created in psychoanalytic treatment principally through the recategorization of memory in the context of the transference.[35] In the broadest sense, psychoanalysis can be thought of as a kind of translation arrived at intersubjectively. Freud suggested that the retranscription of memory is also a kind of translation and that repression, which interferes with *Nachträglichkeit,* represents a refusal to translate.[36] Jean Laplanche, referring to *Nachträglichkeit,* noted Freud's belief that each developmental stratum requires a new translation into a different idiom.[37] *Later developmental epochs provide new meaning for earlier events.* For example, Freud applied the concept of *Nachträglichkeit* to the case of the Wolf Man. The memory of the trauma that the Wolf Man experienced when he witnessed the primal scene at age one and a half was subject to retranscription and endowed with new meaning at age four, and was again translated during his psychoanalysis with Freud at age twenty-four. The essential point is that the meaning of a traumatic event undergoes successive *changes.* Recategorization, which is equivalent to *Nachträglichkeit,* is a *temporal* translation. Anything that interferes with recategorization, such as repression, dissociation, the splitting of the self, or the decentering of the self, results in some loss of freedom.

I have described how trauma interferes with recategorization by preventing the individual from modifying old affect categories in the light of new experiences. Events in real time cannot provide new meaning if the present is interpreted only in terms of the past. If the present cannot modify the past, current events become meaningless. In contrast to people whose lives are dominated by the past, those individuals who lose contact with their affective core lose contact with their past and live in an everlasting present. But this, too, is devoid of meaning. If one does not have access to salient affective memories, the present cannot be recategorized.

As I discussed in *Other Times, Other Realities,* the capacity to experience time as a paradoxical, multileveled reality affords the individual a measure of freedom from the past. This is most evident in assessing a person's capacity to make use of psychoanalytic treatment. Those individuals who can profit most from psychoanalytic treatment are able to experience the paradox of the transference: the relationship with the analyst is perceived both as a repetition of an archaic attachment and as a new relationship. Charles Taylor, in his marvelous work on the conceptual origins of the self, observed that in our modern or postmodern world "there is no single construal of experience which one can cleave to exclusively without disaster or impoverishment"; he concluded that "human life is irreducibly multi-levelled."[38] This observation is illustrated more clearly in art than in science. Taylor cited *The Magic Mountain,* in which Thomas Mann depicted two radically uncombinable modes of the experience of time: the timeless life in the sanatarium and the inescapable intrusion of real events—personal achievements and failures and the outbreak of war.

The complexity of the multileveled consciousness and the multileveled self increases further when one turns to the intersubjective domain. In the social domain, consciousness is multileveled in a different fashion. Instead of a translation from one developmental stratum to the next, as in *Nachträglichkeit,* there is a translation *between* public and private domains.[39] The capacity to enter into the other's experience and yet remain separate enhances the agency of the self and provides the individual with an additional degree of freedom. If one needs to preserve a private construction of reality, if one cannot enter into the experience of others, this places a constraint on one's capacity to learn from others. A hermetic, private construction of reality may help preserve the coherence of the self, but a measure of freedom will have been lost. As we saw in Chapter 4, an infant may be cognitively aware of its separateness, yet its mother's affective synchrony may reinforce a sense of merger with the mother. If this is true, human beings know about paradox at a very early age. It seems to me that the acceptance of paradox is an indicator of mental health.

This multileveled intersubjective consciousness is implicit in Winnicott's *potential space* and Bakhtin's *dialogical mode.*[40] Bakhtin said that in dialogue it is possible to enter into the other through empathy, yet maintain "two nonfused autonomous consciousnesses." Levinas likewise spoke of maintaining the continuity of the self in the presence of the other, and referred to the process as a kind of indwelling, an "at home [*chez soi*] where the self is not altered by the world."[41]

Narrative and the Extension of Meaning

The anthropologist Clifford Geertz made an important observation regarding a current fashion in intellectual life: he noted that in recent years the boundaries between genres have become blurred.[42] Philosophical inquiries may appear in the form of literary criticism, scientific discussions may be presented as belles lettres, and so forth. This trend is also evident in psychoanalysis, where some authors describe the psychoanalytic process as if it were a literary text. Roy Schafer, for example, in his *Retelling a Life,* claims that patients' utterances are texts subject to deconstruction and that psychoanalysis in its entirety can be explained by means of the literary conventions of narrative and dialogue.[43] Even Freud's scientific theories can be viewed, in Schafer's judgment, as a form of narrative. Freud's theories can be seen as a kind of dialogue that alters the patient's text by *destabilizing, deconstructing,* and *defamiliarizing* it.[44]

Schafer has literally disembodied psychoanalysis. It may be useful to consider a patient's construction of his or her life as being analogous to a coherent narrative. But the literary analogy cannot be followed very far, because *the coherence of the psychoanalytic narrative is ultimately derived from the bodily self and its affective memories.* A coherent narrative of one's life does in fact extend the agency of the self. But I suggest that to speak of narrative is simply to emphasize the temporal—that is, the historical—nature of the self. In *Time and Narrative* Paul Ricoeur said, "Time becomes human to the extent that it is articulated through a narrative mode," and maintained that narration is an imitation of life which is reconfigured through time.[45] *Language acquires a temporal dimension through narrative.*[46] Temporality is brought to language to the extent that language (through narrative) figures and refigures temporal experience. The narrative mode always implies a certain reconfiguration of time.[47]

Jerome Bruner, in *Acts of Meaning,* likewise emphasizes the central function of narrative in the extension of meaning.[48] Although Bruner believes, as I do, that the agency of the self is inseparable from the construction of meaning, he focuses nearly exclusively upon the acquisition of meaning through cultural narratives and therefore minimizes the significance of the creation of private meanings. He appears to lean in the direction of those social theorists who emphasize the social self at the expense of the private self. For example, citing the series *A History of Private Life,* Bruner reports with apparent approval that "privacy is to be understood as a 'spin-off' from post-medieval sociopolitical arrangements rather than an expression of some basic psychological or biological need."[49]

We are very far from understanding the relation between privately created narratives and culturally imposed narratives. But it is reasonable to suppose that since narrative dictates some coherent temporal order, it contributes to the sense of coherence of self. Finally, it should be noted that the narrative mode is only one means among many of achieving this coherence of self. The lesson to be learned from neurobiology is that we must allow for an enormous variety of individual differences.

I consider the coherence and continuity of the self to be a fundamental biological value, a homeostat. A homeostat is defined as a system that maintains the conditions necessary for life. I am aware that my perspective on the self is undeniably formed by Western culture, as Charles Taylor has so ably demonstrated. If I were an Indian or a Japanese psychoanalyst, my discussion of the agency of the self would undoubtedly take a different form. In the West there is an emphasis on agency as self actualization. I have suggested that this sense of personal effectiveness contributes to the feeling of coherence and continuity of the self. In non-Western cultures such a sense of coherence may be achieved by other means. The sense of coherence and continuity may be achieved through one's role in the family and in the larger society. In non-Western culture the coherence of the self seems to be provided for by a transpersonal awareness. Sudhir Kakar, an Indian psychoanalyst, suggests that the idea of separateness and individuality is a Western value.[50] In India the emphasis is on the transpersonal nature of man: the body is considered to have intimate connections with nature and the cosmos. This cultural relativism does not, I believe, negate the biological thesis that pervades this book. Given the enormous biological diversity of individuals, the diversity of cultures is not in itself an argument for nurture as opposed to nature.

Summary

The process of psychoanalysis extends the agency of the self through the creation of new meanings. "Meaning," in the lexicon of psychoanalysts, denotes personal—that is, private—meaning. This contrasts with the usage of some linguists and philosophers of language, whose concern is the understanding of public and shared meanings. In this chapter I have marshaled some of the evidence for the embodiment of meaning. This differentiates my position from that of researchers who see meaning in psychoanalysis as analogous to a literary text; for I believe that what is meaningful in psychoanalysis can ultimately be traced to affective memories. The psychoanalyst can observe embodied meaning, since a patient's communication is meaningful only if it carries with it some affective charge. The coherence of the psychoanalytic narrative is ultimately derived from the bodily self and its affective memories. This embodiment of meaning is supported by Edelman's theory of Neuronal Group

Selection, particularly his concept of evolutionary values that exert a selective influence upon perception.

The coherence of the self is enhanced through the creation of new meanings, and this process in turn requires that memories be recategorized. Identifying the ideational content of affects and naming affects also facilitate a sense of agency.

Trauma can be brought within the agency of the self through the creation of new meanings. I have interpreted Freud's account of his grandson's *fort-da* game from this perspective.

The process of psychoanalysis provides an opportunity to observe the interplay between private and shared meanings, as evidenced in the patient's and analyst's constructions of reality. The developmental effect of marked divergences between the child's and the adult's constructions of reality may impair the child's ability to learn from others. Such divergent constructions of reality regularly occur in cases where the child is sexually abused by an adult and in other forms of traumatic interactions.

The creation of new meanings through recategorization affords the individual a certain degree of freedom from the domination of the past. This, in turn, is facilitated if there is a capacity to experience consciousness on more than one level.

8

Value, "Instinct," and the Emergent Motives of the Self

> How odd it is that anyone should not see that all observation must be for or against some view if it is to be of any service!
> CHARLES DARWIN, letter to Henry Fawcett

> It is much easier to formulate a theory of psychology which simply neglects the difficult questions concerning the relationship of psychology to neurology.
> ROBERT SOLOMON, "Freud's Neurological Theory of Mind"

In this chapter, we shall look at the crisis of contemporary psychoanalytic theory that has resulted from Freud's antiquated psychobiology, and shall focus on the biological matrix of the private self—the premise that the need to maintain the continuity and coherence of the self is a homeostatic function. We shall see that a biological theory of value is a promising substitute for an anachronistic instinct theory.

Contemporary psychoanalytic theory has lost its central organizing principle. To use Kuhn's terms, it has lost its "paradigm."[1] As Kuhn observed, a scientific theory is declared invalid only if an alternative candidate is available to take its place. The psychology of the self has been proposed as an alternative to current psychoanalytic theory, but its own fundamental conceptual categories are not easy to discern. Analytic theory today comes in many versions: classical or neoclassical (sometimes called structural) theory, object relations theory, self psychology, interpersonal or relational theory, Kleinian theory, Lacanian theory, and so forth. It is evident that Freud's theoretical edifice has lost its conceptual glue.

I suggest that the conceptual crisis in contemporary psychoanalytic theory has two principal root causes. First, Freud's instinct theory, the foundation stone of the psychoanalytic edifice, is incongruent with contemporary biology. Second, the psychology of the self encompasses emergent motivations of a very different conceptual order from Freud's conception of instinct. I distinguish "motivation" from "agency." These terms overlap to some extent, but "agency" as applied to the self usually connotes a degree of conscious mastery, whereas motivations can be both conscious and unconscious.

Since the energy of Freud's mental apparatus is derived from instinct, this leads to the question of how impersonal instincts such as sexuality and aggression can become transformed into personal motives. How does the self—or, in Freud's language, the ego—put its personal imprint on an instinct? Freud would answer that a private sexual wish, fantasy, or feeling is a *representation* of the libidinal instinct. But this explanation places too great a burden on the concept of representation, which must explain how an impersonal impulse (a physiological need) is transformed into a meaningful wish.

This conceptual problem—impersonal energy versus the personal wish—has been a divisive issue within psychoanalysis for several decades. I am among those psychoanalysts who believe that the ultimate motivating agency is not the id or the ego but the self. Those who recognize the self as a superordinate agent, however, are divided as to whether that agent, the self, is embodied or disembodied. For those who consider the agency of the self to be outside biology must also consider psychoanalytic theory to be outside biology.

Kohut, Schafer, and Lacan, who have emphasized the primacy of the agency of the self, have all viewed psychoanalysis as disembodied. In his last paper, Kohut emphasized that he was motivated to develop his theory of self psychology because he was so opposed to the drive concept, which he saw as the intrusion of a "vague and insipid biological concept into a marvelous system of psychology." He similarly dismissed the concepts of dependence, autonomy, identity, and adaptation as "intrusions imported from social psychology."[2] Although *identity* is socially bestowed, the continuity of the self, which is dependent upon memory, is clearly a biological concept, as are *dependence, autonomy,* and *adaptation.* Kohut described intense rage and intense lust as "disintegration products" of the self. I understand him to mean that when rage and lust are disruptive, they can be viewed as products of the failure of the agency of the self. It would perhaps be more accurate to speak of a relative failure of the transformational capacities of the self. In Kohut's formulation, the self watches helplessly as it is replaced by experience over which it has no influence or control. But it is difficult for me to follow the logic of Kohut's claim that such a process places the self outside biology.

This debate within psychoanalysis is paralleled by a similar debate within neuroscience, cognitive science, and philosophy. There is a sharp division between those who assert that the brain, and by implication the mind, are a supercomplex information processing machine and those who believe that the brain (and the mind) can be understood only in the context of evolutionary biology. Edelman has extensively reviewed this controversy in his book *Bright Air, Brilliant Fire.*[3]

Lacan, who also rejected a biology of the self, believed that at the time the infant is weaned it passes from the biological domain into the world of language and culture. Lacan claimed that because psychoanalysis operates within the mode of speech and language, it is a "mental" science, allied more closely to sociology and anthropology than to biology. As Malcolm Bowie has noted, Lacan interpreted the psychoanalyst's biological explanations as fantasies, as evidence of the *psychoanalyst's* wish to return to a state prior to weaning, a state of merger with the mother.[4] As we noted earlier, Ruth Millikan has demonstrated that language is not something outside biology, for language is a normative function, itself a product of evolutionary history. Contrast this view with that of Roy Schafer in his book *A New Language for Psychoanalysis.* He argued that "action language" should replace the "biological language of functions which cannot be concerned with meaning" and asked, "What can a mindless instinctual drive have to do with a phenomenal thought?"[5] Later, in *The Analytic Attitude*[6] and *Retelling a Life,*[7] Schafer emphasized the overriding significance of a disembodied narrative. But narration is only one way of creating meaning and safeguarding the coherence of the self. The emergent value of self coherence is more salient, and each individual safeguards the coherence of the self in his or her own fashion.

Evolutionary Biology and the Fall of Instinct Theory

There is considerable difference of opinion within psychoanalysis as to whether Freud was in fact a "biologist of the mind."[8] There are those who claim that in his "Project for a Scientific Psychology" and his book *On Aphasia,* Freud used the language of neurophysiology to clothe his essentially psychological theories—that his theories were not primarily neurophysiological and that he used neurophysiology only as a metaphor to shape his essentially psychological model of the mind.[9] I do not agree with this interpretation, but the issue is debatable. What I consider beyond debate is the evident fact that Freud grounded his theory of instincts in evolutionary biology. In this he did not waver. Freud mistakenly believed that experience over long periods of time could be inherited and that evolutionary processes affected primarily the fitness of the group rather than the fitness of the individual.[10] "There is naturally nothing to prevent our supposing that the instincts themselves are, at least in part, precipitates of the effect of external stimulation, which in the course of phylogenesis have brought about modifications in the living substance."[11] Freud's belief in Lamarckianism, his uncritical acceptance of Haeckel's law that ontogeny recapitulates phylogeny, and his misunderstanding of population theory were all commonplace in the late nineteenth and early twentieth centuries.[12]

Freud also made it evident that he relied on biology for his psychoanalytic classification of instincts. He originally suggested the existence of two superordinate instincts, ego instincts and sexual instincts, and stated that this distinction could not be based on psychological considerations alone.[13] Libido theory derives its principal support from biology.[14] Freud noted that it would be desirable to keep psychology clear of everything different from it, including biology, but that this was not possible.[15] He supported his differentiation of the ego instincts (self preservation) from the sexual instincts by referring to Weismann's concept of the germ-plasm. In Freud's view, the conflict between sexual desire and self preservation reflected a deeper conflict in nature: that between the transitory need for the survival of the individual and the more lasting requirement of the survival of the species. He recognized, however, that this classification of instincts was provisional and would inevitably be modified by advances in biology. With his final classification of instincts as eros and thanatos in "Beyond the Pleasure Principle," he admitted the uncertainty of his speculations—an uncertainty that was increased by the need to borrow from biology: "Biology is a land of unlimited possibilities. We cannot guess what answers it will return in a few dozen years. They may be of a kind that will blow away the whole of our artificial structure of our hypotheses."[16]

Some may object that this discussion of evolutionary biology is misleading because Freud was referring not to instincts but to *drive,* and because Strachey arbitrarily translated *Trieb* as "instinct."[17] Jean Laplanche and J.-B. Pontalis observed that the word *Trieb* is derived from *treiben,* meaning "to push"; hence the term "drive."[18] It should also be acknowledged that Freud did distinguish *Instinkt,* a rigid behavioral pattern seen in animals, from *Trieb.* He used the term *Instinkt* to refer to behavior that is virtually identical in all members of the same species. Freud did not believe, however, that *Trieb*—in contrast to *Instinkt*—could be thought of as a purely psychological concept, for he never indicated that *Trieb* could be considered outside an evolutionary context: "If we now apply ourselves to considering mental life from a *biological* point of view, an 'instinct' appears to us as a concept on the frontier between the mental and the somatic, as the psychical representative of the stimuli originating from within the organism and reaching the mind, as a measure of the demand made upon the mind for work in consequence of its connection with the body."[19]

But although Freud acknowledged the conceptual precariousness of the instinct concept and the provisional nature of his classification of instincts, the dual instinct theory remained as an elementary and fundamental psychoanalytic tenet. I believe that for Freud, "instinct" corresponded to those basic theoretical entities upon which a theory rests, analogous to the physicist's elementary particles. As he himself wrote, "Psychoanalysis early became aware that *all mental occurrences must be regarded as built on the basis of an interplay of forces of the elementary instincts.*"[20] Instinct theory provided the explanation for both intrapsychic conflict and the conflict that exists between the individual and society. According to Hans Loewald, Freud believed that the id (the repository of instincts) was the ultimate psychic reality.[21]

The interpretive power of instinct theory was indeed impressive. Not only did instinct explain motivation; it also explained the ubiquity of intrapsychic conflict as a derivative of the battle between eros and thanatos. Positing an instinctual origin for wishes and fantasies provided an explanation for a broad range of clinical phenomena, from character disorders to schizophrenia. These conditions could be explained by postulating a fixation or regression of instinctual development.[22] Karl Abraham, for example, linked the oral phase to schizophrenia and depression and the anal phase to obsessive compulsive disorders.[23] He observed that those individuals with an obsessive compulsive neurosis evidenced an exaggerated interest in possessing and retaining objects, as well as a peculiar ambivalence regarding orderliness and cleanliness.

The theory of instincts provided an analogy to geology, by allowing phenomena to be classified in accordance with their developmental strata. In this sense, instinct theory made a psychoanalytic archeology possible, because fantasies and wishes could be classified developmentally. Instinctual phenomena could be described not only along a developmental axis, but along other axes as well. Instincts could be characterized as active or passive and, furthermore, could be characterized according to the degree to which eros was combined with hatred. These axes could be used as descriptive grids describing and classifying the wishes and fantasies that motivate behavior. Fantasies and wishes could be described as oral receptive, oral sadistic, anal retentive, anal sadistic, and so forth. Passive phallic exhibitionism could be distinguished from active phallic sadism and, in turn, both could be differentiated from true genitality. The Oedipus complex was seen as the confluence and culmination of libido theory, and, accordingly, psychoanalytic chronology strictly separated the oedipal from the pre-oedipal. Given the sweep and power of this theory, one can understand why many psychoanalysts have fought hard to preserve the paradigm.

As we have noted, a change of paradigm requires an alternative theory, and the theory of the self has been proposed as such an alternative. But the paradoxical nature of the self—as both an abiding structure and an ephemeral experience—has led to disjunctive theories. For example, we have on the one hand Fairbairn's structural conception of the self as internalized object relationships and, on the other, Kohut's phenomenological self psychology. Both Fairbairn and Kohut denied the validity of Freud's instinct theory, but neither offered alternative concepts covering the phenomena that instinct theory explained. Fairbairn's consideration of impulses as energized structures is too general and abstract, and Kohut dismissed instincts as "disintegration products" of the self.

It is only within the latter half of the twentieth century that studies of the evolution of behavior developed into a separate discipline; in this process, the term "instinct" lost its scientific status.[24] I do not know exactly when this occurred. In a 1935 article Konrad Lorenz, recognized as the founder of ethology, accepted the validity of instinct as a concept.[25] But if one consults more recent authoritative texts on the evolution of behavior, one discovers that the term "instinct" (or "drive") hardly exists.[26] Edward Wilson, in his influential survey of the evolution of behavior, pays scant attention to the concept of instinct and does little more than repeat the conventional definition of "instinct" as genetically determined behavior that is subject to relatively little modification as a result of experience.[27] In a more fundamental sense the concept of instinct is no longer sustainable, because it is what Ernst Mayr has termed an "essentialist" concept—that is, a "God's-Eye View."[28] If instinct is a product of evolution, it cannot be a uniform entity corresponding to a Platonic essence, since evolution selects for individual variations in a population of unique individuals. Instinct and species must both be thought of as *selectionist* concepts.[29]

The problem with the concept of instinct was addressed by Gregory Bateson, who in response to the question "What is an instinct?" said, "It is a label for what a certain black box is supposed to do."[30] Bateson viewed the term "instinct" as a nonexplanation, a word coined before anyone knew anything about genetics, a word which is very difficult to translate into modern ideas. With regard to evolutionary biology, the concept "instinct" appears to have joined the ranks of pseudoexplanations such as phlogiston. It would be ironic if psychoanalysis, once a revolutionary discipline, became the preserve of obsolete scientific concepts. This does not mean, however, that we can ignore what the term "instinct" signified. Instead, evolutionary biologists refer to "functional motivational systems." From the standpoint of contemporary studies of the evolution of behavior, there is no such entity as an instinct for self preservation. There are instead behaviors that are selected and that enhance the fitness of the individual.

Object relations theorists such as Winnicott, Loewald, and John Bowlby have questioned Freud's instinct theory from another direction. They all challenge Freud's view that the object of instinct is simply that through which the instinct achieves its aim.[31] The *object* in Freud's earlier concept of instinct was not a person but an erogenous zone.

Bowlby, using ethological evidence, demonstrated a very close correspondence between attachment behavior in primates and attachment behavior in the human child.[32] In all primate species so far investigated, separation of a child from its mother causes anxiety and what can be interpreted as grief. Bowlby made the important point that attachment behavior and sexuality are separate motivational systems. Attachment behavior ensures the survival and safety of the immature individual by making relatedness a value; the bond of relatedness between the mother and her offspring is safeguarded by the fact that both offspring and mother experience anxiety upon separation. For the infant, loss is signaled through separation anxiety; for the mother, attachment behavior is motivated by what Winnicott called "primary maternal preoccupation."[33] All of these behaviors are manifestations of evolutionary "values" (in Edelman's use of that term). Attachment behavior, unlike sexuality, is not orgastic or tension reducing; it moves silently.[34]

Psychoanalytic Reinterpretations of Freud's Concept of Instinct

Bowlby's contribution demonstrated that attachment behavior is an evolutionary given, a system of values that is part of our phenotype. Therefore, if something approximating Freud's classification of instinct were to be maintained, it would have to include attachment behavior. Then it would be a trilogy of instincts and not a duality.

Winnicott's claim that there is no such thing as an infant covers the same ground as Bowlby's notion of attachment behavior. Winnicott spoke of an "ego relatedness" that takes precedence over the forces of the id.[35] For example, Winnicott described some mothers who, instead of relating to their infants, "fob them off" with a feed.[36]

Loewald reinterpreted Freud's instinct concept as a process, not an entity: "instincts, understood as psychic, motivational forces, become organized as such through interactions with a psychic field consisting originally of the mother-child (psychic) unit."[37] Although Loewald believed that he remained faithful to Freud's instinct theory, it seems to me that he radically transformed Freud's concept of instinct. Instead of viewing instincts as fixed entities, he treated them as a process formed in interaction with the environment: the environment "engenders and organizes excitation processes."[38] Loewald's view of instinct is, as we shall see, consistent with Edelman's neurobiological concept of an evolutionary value modified by reentry—that is, modified by experience.

The Frontier between Psychoanalysis and Biology

If evolutionary biology can no longer support the concept of instinctual entities, and if the concept of instinct or drive is essential for psychoanalytic theory, one way of resolving this impasse is to assert, as Loewald has, that the concept of drive or instinct is not a biological concept but a *psychoanalytic concept*.[39] Jay Greenberg has attempted to expand Loewald's position that the psychoanalytic concept of instinct is a psychological concept and not necessarily a biological concept; he considers the embodiment of psychoanalysis to be only a "strategy," a theoretical option.[40]

If instinct were considered entirely a psychological concept, it would no longer be on the frontier—on the border, as Freud said, between body and mind. I am reminded here of Robert Solomon's dictum that appears at the head of this chapter: it is much easier to formulate a theory of psychology which neglects the difficult question concerning the relationship of psychology to the brain.[41]

In considering the frontier between biology and psychoanalysis, one returns again to the fundamental question of the relation of mind to brain. Freud's position was ambiguous, in that he both retained and rejected a Cartesian duality. That Freud believed in the unity of mind and brain is evidenced in his continued conviction that psychic energy is not a metaphor but a literal manifestation of a neuronal state. But he was not consistent. For in his monograph on aphasia (a section of which is reprinted in "The Unconscious")[42] Freud accepted the conventional wisdom of Hughlings Jackson and stated that "the psychical is a process parallel to the physiological"—a "dependent concomitant." Perhaps Freud was unwilling to advertise his radical departure from the "scientific" Cartesian view. At any rate, despite Freud's inconsistency, Solomon views him as a monist on the mind-brain issue.[43] It has also been suggested that Freud's inconsistency and his use of multiple models and mixed metaphors are a virtue when dealing with the enormously complex concepts on the frontier between mind and body.[44]

Another argument for the disembodiment of psychoanalysis is that to confuse the mind with the brain is tantamount to reducing psychoanalysis to neurobiology. For example, Edelson states that "nonphysical" sciences such as

psychoanalysis are autonomous in the same sense that sociology, anthropology, and economics are autonomous.[45] For
this reason, Edelson claims that psychoanalysis cannot be
replaced or reduced by neuroscience. Those who warn of
the dangers of reductionism usually point to the excesses of
some sociobiologists who believed that certain cultural phenomena could be "explained" by genetics. In *Bright Air,
Brilliant Fire,* Edelman argues against what he calls "silly"
reductionism—the belief that neuroscience will reduce the
human spirit to molecules or synapses. All sciences are autonomous, yet must share concepts that lie across their frontiers. Every discipline needs to create its own concepts and
terminology in accordance with its special field of observation and theoretical requirements. In this sense every discipline is autonomous, but the autonomy is only relative and
not absolute.[46] As there are many levels of conceptualization
within a given discipline, there are also many shared borders. For example, psychoanalysis shares borders with the
social sciences as well as with cognitive science and neurobiology. Philip Holzman and Gerald Aronson have urged
that psychoanalysts ally themselves with these scientific
neighbors.[47]

In contrast to those psychoanalysts who claim that biology
has no place in psychoanalysis, there are perhaps just as
many who have repeatedly and consistently affirmed psychoanalysis' ties to biology.[48] I am not prepared to review the
work of all of the psychoanalysts who have reaffirmed that
tie. But we should at least make note of Heinz Hartmann,
whose well-known monograph *Ego Psychology and the Problem of Adaptation* is essentially an essay in applied biology.
John Gedo's hierarchical model of the mind reflects the body's
hierarchical organization.[49] Fred Levin has used Gedo's hierarchical model to attempt a synthesis of neurobiology and psy-

choanalysis.[50] And Morton Reiser, in a series of volumes, has demonstrated the links between psychoanalysis and neurobiology.[51]

Value and a Theory of the Emergent Motives of the Self

As Hilary Putnam noted, words, concepts, and categories—like individuals—have their own history.[52] The term "instinct" had a history as a concept in folk psychology before it became a scientific term. We are gradually recognizing the extent to which our folk concepts and categories have been influenced by certain philosophical assumptions, which then become tacit assumptions behind scientific concepts.[53] One such assumption is that a category, such as instinct, corresponds to a Platonic essentialist ideal. The essentialist ideal assumes that a category contains certain properties which make it what it is: a uniform entity, a thing in itself defined by its "essence." Ernst Mayr has emphasized that the pre-Darwinian idea of what constitutes a species is an essentialist (Platonic) concept. Mayr distinguished the typologist from the population thinker: "For the typologist, the type *(eidos)* is real and the variation an illusion, while for the populationist the type is an abstraction and only the variation is real."[54] Darwin himself used the term "instinct" but intended that it denote behavior reflecting an evolutionary selectionist process rather than an entity.

Edelman's theory of Neuronal Group Selection provides a means of escaping from the essentialist concept of instinct. The term "value" is sufficiently inclusive that it can extend from the organism's homeostatic systems to the domain of personal interests and personal meanings. *Value is therefore a border-crossing concept that spans the mind and the brain.* "Value," referring to evolutionary constraints, exerts a bias upon the process of reentry so that *genetic constraints are both intercalated with and transformed by an epigenetic developmental process.* For example, when one considers sexuality as a motivational system, there are genetic givens that exist side by side with epigenetic transformations. This abstract statement may be concretized if we consider the example of homosexuality. Psychoanalysis has long recognized the basic distinction between homosexuality as a fundamental preference (which neuroscience may show to be genetic) and a homosexual choice which is reactive or defensive— which may be at variance with the individual's physiological heterosexuality but which can be understood in the context of his or her developmental history.

As Edelman has underscored, value combined with reentry leads to new selectional properties.[55] This means that motivational systems are not only genetically constrained but also *emergent.* This point is especially relevant for the emergent motivations of the self that I have been emphasizing throughout this work: the self is a creator of meaning, value, and interests. In Chapter 2 I described the joy that young children experience in mastery—a joy that has been called the "pleasure of efficacy." This motivational system is not orgastic and has nothing to do with tension reduction, yet it unquestionably represents an evolutionary value that is emergent. There are many other emergent values associated with the self which can be thought of as powerful motivational systems—passionate interests, for example. Passionate interests affirm the coherence of the self: some people will willingly die for what they believe.

Briefly, Edelman's theory of Neuronal Group Selection proposes that *selective processes favoring adaptation occur at the level of neuronal groups during individual development, from conception onward. A dynamic selective process occurs in these neuronal groups in somatic time (that is, from conception to death). This selective process in somatic time is competitive, in the sense that it favors certain synaptic connections over others, so that an analogous process that Darwin described in evolutionary time occurs within neuronal groups in somatic time.*[56]

Darwinian selection requires diversity. Neural Darwinism proposes that such a selective process operating upon neuronal groups likewise requires diversity. Such diversity is present anatomically and physiologically (identical twins do not have identical brains). But diversity is also created by the brain itself when *value is combined with reentry*.

Edelman introduced the term "value" to denote those evolutionary constraints favoring behavior that fulfills homeostatic requirements or contributes to the inclusive fitness of the organism. "Reentry" refers to the global coordination of sensory inputs that is necessary to account for the individual's spatio-temporal continuity, and by implication the continuity and coherence of the self. *Value acts as a bias on reentry.*

Value as an evolutionary constraint should not be confused with that which is unlearned. Rather, such constraints direct or select that which is of *interest* to the individual—select what is to be learned. Value exerts a selective influence on experience. As Konrad Lorenz wrote, "In regard to behavior, *the innate is not only what is not learned, but what must be in existence before all individual learning to make learning possible.*"[57] With the concepts of value and reentry, the ancient dichotomy between nature and nurture cannot be maintained.

The Continuity and Coherence of the Self as a Homeostat

The need to maintain the continuity and coherence of the self is a vital urge of no less importance than sexual desire or the need for attachment to others. I propose that the continuity and coherence of the self is such a psychobiological homeostat.[58] It is a transcendent value that is congruent with the global functions of the brain. This was implied by Kurt Goldstein, who asserted that there is only one motive by which human activity is initiated:[59] the tendency to actualize oneself.[60] The OED defines "coherence" as the act of cleaving or sticking together. Observations of infants suggest that coherence of self is supported by an unconscious synchrony between infants and their caretakers. As Winnicott put it, "the mother keeps time going for the infant."[61] It seems that coherence and continuity are mutually reinforcing loops: the "sticking together" of the self reinforces its continuity, and vice versa. This intersubjective synchrony is gradually internalized by the child but never completely internalized. Adults retain this need for intersubjective synchrony, which Kohut described as the continuing need for a selfobject. This may also take the form of a self-created presence or muse (as we saw in Chapter 5). However, we know that since the coherence of the self is dependent upon another person, this process is double-edged. For beyond infancy there is a biologically determined divergence of need between the caretaker and the child.[62] This is reflected in their divergent constructions of reality.[63] In the older child and in the adult, the coherence of the self becomes less dependent on others, since it is largely self created through language and through the construction of personal narratives,[64] moral commitments, and passionate interests. The philosopher Irving Singer, in *Meaning in Life,* suggests that meaning *in* life (as distinct from the meaning *of* life) rests upon the emergence of self-created values, interests, and imaginative acts. For those who retain a belief in God, there is a ready-made sense of one's place in the universe—a sense that contributes to the coherence of the self. Conversely, in the absence of such beliefs there is a greater strain placed upon the self in order to maintain this sense of coherence.[65]

Hull, as he tells us in his autobiography, *Touching the Rock,* struggled to reestablish the coherence of his self following the loss of his sight. He describes how he gradually abandoned his interest in visual meaning in favor of other values that the self creates:

"As one goes deeper and deeper into blindness the things which once were taken for granted, and which were then mourned over when they disappeared, and for which one tried in various ways to find compensation, in the end cease to matter. Somehow, it no longer seems important what people look like or what cities look like. One cannot check first hand the accuracy of these reports, they lose personal meaning and are relegated to the edge of awareness. They become irrelevant in the conduct of one's life. One begins to live by other interests, other values. One begins to take up residence in another world."[66]

Winnicott proposed that the maternal holding environment assured the infant's continuity of being.[67] Some children discover that they must protect the private self from intrusions that disturb the sense of continuity. The task of maintaining continuity and coherence then falls on the private self, which can create, through imagination, its own protective presences, although it cannot accomplish this in complete isolation. Other values will emerge as a selective bias which reinforces those actions that preserve continuity and coherence. The joy of self actualization, whether experienced by a child learning to walk or by an artist in the act of creation, demonstrates the inherent pleasure that is released by acts that reinforce the coherence and continuity of the self.[68] This is different from the pleasure of "orgastic release" and cannot be explained as an instinctual "sublimation."[69]

As is true of most homeostats, whenever a steady state is threatened with interruption the individual experiences signals of danger—warnings to restore the equilibrium. Here the primordial signal of danger is that of the disintegration of the self: annihilation anxiety. (One need only think of William James, who feared that his self could be transformed into the pitiable patient he once viewed in an asylum.) Most of us do not experience this ultimate anxiety because automatic, unconscious defensive processes forestall such an eventuality. As is often the case, the defensive process itself may become a new form of pathology. From a neurobiological perspective, this defensive reaction to trauma will disrupt what Edelman calls "higher-order consciousness," an ability to maintain a model of past, present, and future.

The self is a paradox—both ephemeral and continuous. I have suggested that Edelman's concepts of reentry and recategorization go a long way toward resolving that paradox. For reentry and recategorization provide a sense of continuity in the face of the discontinuities of the physical world. The capacity to recategorize memory seems to be the basis for the continuity of time, the continuity of the self.

One may object that the term "value" is overly inclusive. I have suggested that the continuity and coherence of the self is a value encompassing both mind and brain. Furthermore, "value" denotes aspects of human motivation that are genetically constrained and shared by the species, as well as emergent aspects of the self, such as the joy of effective actions and passionate interests that are not genetically constrained but highly individualized and plastic. This coexistence or intercalation of that which is genetically constrained on the one hand and developmentally emergent and plastic on the other has been noted by Freud and others. For this reason, Freud made a distinction between *Instinkt* and *Trieb*. Robert Hinde, in his synthesis of ethology and comparative psychology, suggested that it is useful to characterize items of behavior in accordance with their stability or lability under environmental influences.[70] Thus, Silvan Tomkins differentiated drives from affects.[71] He reasoned that a drive such as hunger is relatively constrained (genetically), yet a baby's cry has a multitude of causes. He contrasted the relative fixity of drives with the variability of affects, and concluded that drives have motivational impact only when amplified by affects.

We may, therefore, need to differentiate values that are relatively constrained from those that are highly emergent. But if we accept Edelman's concept that value exerts a bias on reentry, it is no longer possible to maintain a clear distinction between what is genetic and what is epigenetic.

Freud returned to the relation between the genetically constrained elements and the more plastic elements in personality in his 1937 paper "Analysis Terminable and Interminable."[72] He believed that the innate strength of instinct and the "innate distinguishing characteristics of the ego" predispose the individual to choose one type of defense over another. For these reasons, Freud offered a pessimistic note of caution regarding the therapeutic efficacy of psychoanalysis. I would include these factors under the category of genetic restraints. Though I do not question Freud's caution, he might have been more optimistic had he known that neuroscience would demonstrate that neural events and hence mental events are unpredictable. He may have recognized that with uncertainty, there is no linear progression between the strength of instincts and pathological outcome. With uncertainty, it is possible to devise new and highly individualized solutions that are not necessarily pathological.

Summary

I have traced the conceptual crisis in psychoanalytic theory to two principal root causes. First, instinct theory is incongruent with contemporary evolutionary biology. Second, the psychology of the self encompasses emergent motivations of a very different conceptual order from that of instinct theory.

One response to this conceptual crisis has been the disembodiment of psychoanalysis. The agency of the self, and psychoanalysis as a whole, are viewed by many psychoanalytic authors as outside biology. There are other psychoanalysts who wish to preserve Freud's instinct theory by asserting that instinct or drive is a psychoanalytic and not a biological concept.

I have offered an alternative proposal, suggesting that Gerald Edelman's neurobiological theory of evolutionary value can potentially substitute for the discredited concept of instinct. The term "value" is sufficiently inclusive that it can extend from the organism's homeostatic systems to the domain of personal interests and personal meanings. "Value" is therefore a border-crossing concept that spans mind and brain and provides biological backing for a theory of emergent motives of the self.

The homeostasis of the self, expressed as a need to maintain coherence and continuity, is a vital urge of no less importance than sexual desire or the need for attachment to others. In adult life the coherence and continuity of the self becomes less dependent on others because it is largely self created through moral commitments and passionate interests, as well as through the assimilation and construction of personal and social narratives.

The concept of value includes that which is genetically constrained, as well as emergent properties that are more variable and plastic. This was a subject that Freud considered in his paper "Analysis Terminable and Interminable." Freud's pessimism regarding the inevitable pathological outcome of genetic constraints, such as the strength of the instincts and the deformations of the ego, would have been modified had he known that neuroscience would demonstrate the indeterminacy and unpredictability of neural events. Indeterminacy justifies a certain therapeutic hopefulness. In a larger sense, we may also hope that contemporary neuroscience will help reestablish the Freudian vision of the unity of psyche and soma, of the unity of mind and brain.

Notes

In cases where two editions of a particular work are cited in the references, the page numbers given in the notes refer to the later edition.

1. Thinking about the Self

1. Levinas 1961, p. 36.
2. Lichtenstein 1961. This point will be discussed in Chapter 8.
3. For further discussion of this point see Fine 1990.
4. Grossman 1982; Hume 1739, p. 229, emphasis added.
5. Nozick 1981.
6. Winnicott 1962.
7. Freud 1917, p. 249.
8. Erikson 1959, p. 113.
9. Lichtenstein (1963, p. 199) notes the paradoxical nature of identity. "Identity as experience of the pure actuality of being remains indefinable, unworldly. Any definable identity requires that we perceive ourselves as objects, which means equating identity with the identity given to us as social roles, thereby losing the sense of identity as pure actuality of being."
10. Federn 1952.
11. Freud 1923, p. 17.
12. Freud 1926.
13. Taylor 1989, p. 175.
14. Draenos 1982; Lear 1990.
15. Solomon (1974, p. 35) commented on this problem as follows: "The model of the psychic apparatus is essentially a theory of the *Other*. Accordingly, psychological predicates are not first person observation reports but rather theoretical terms that serve a function in an

overall theory of human behavior and psychology." Solomon observed that Freud substituted a methodological dualism for a metaphysical dualism.

16. Grossman and Simon (1969), as well as Nagel (1974), suggest that Freud's anthropomorphisms should not be dismissed. Grossman and Simon indicate that Freud's anthropomorphism is not only inevitable when one attempts to report the results of introspection but also necessary as a means of organizing experience. These authors also cite Freud's comment about anthropomorphism: "It is not at all necessary to outgrow it. Our understanding reaches as far as our anthropomorphisms."

17. Freud 1921, p. 130.

18. Freud 1940, p. 205, emphasis added.

19. Freud 1923, p. 58.

20. Ibid., p. 54.

21. Hartmann, Kris, and Loewenstein 1946; Hartmann 1956.

22. For further discussion of Freud's ambiguity concerning the distinction between self and ego, see Spruiell 1981; Kernberg 1982; Modell 1984.

23. The *International Review of Psychoanalysis* recently devoted an entire issue to this subject; see *International Review of Psychoanalysis* 18, part 3 (1991). In this debate Strachey also has his defenders, such as Laplanche (1991), who discusses the difficulties of translating colloquial language into the more specialized usage of psychoanalysis. For other comments on Strachey's translations, see Ornston 1982, 1985, 1985a; Kernberg 1982; and McIntosh 1986.

24. Gilman 1990.

25. *Besetzung* is a German term that has no precise English equivalent. In Austria it is a frequently used word that varies in accordance with its context but is generally understood to mean "taking something over and using it in a certain way" (Ornston 1985b).

26. Faimberg 1988.

27. Fairbairn 1952.

28. It is of interest to note that he retained the term "libido" while rejecting the concept of instinct.

29. Fairbairn 1952, pp. 33, 85.

30. Sutherland 1989.

31. This and other traumatic episodes in Fairbairn's childhood were reconstructed by means of interviews with family members and close associates; see Dawson 1985.

32. Fairbairn 1952, p. 105.

33. Fairbairn's emphasis on the internalization of relationships that form a core of the self corresponds to current observation of infants. Stern (1985) asserts that an early core of the sense of self consists of "representations of interactions that have become generalized." See also Beebe and Lachmann 1988.

34. Fairbairn's dialogue with Freud is discussed in Modell 1968, 1975; Greenberg and Mitchell 1983; and Hughes 1989.

35. Sutherland 1989, p. 147.

36. Stern 1985.

37. Fairbairn 1952, p. 107.

38. Ibid., p. 159.

39. See Chasseguet-Smirgel 1985 for an extensive discussion of the difference between the ego ideal and the superego.

40. Perhaps the clearest illustration of the extent to which Freud was influenced by Haeckel can be seen in his recently discovered work *A Phylogenetic Fantasy* (Freud 1987).

41. Freud 1923, p. 38.

42. Freud 1933, p. 64.

43. Kernberg 1976.

44. Bollas 1987.

45. Ibid., p. 58.

46. Hartmann 1950.

47. Ibid., p. 85.

48. Freud 1915a, p. 213: "The object-presentation itself is once again a complex of associations made up of the greatest variety of visual, acoustic, tactile, kinaesthetic and other presentations. Philosophy tells us that an object-presentation consists of nothing more than this—that the appearance of there being a 'thing' to whose various 'attributes' these sense impressions bear witness is merely due to the fact that, in enumerating the sense-impressions which we have received from an object, we also assume the possibility of there being a

large number of further sense impressions in the same chain of associations." (Freud is here citing J. S. Mill.) Apparently Freud used the term "representation" in several different contexts. He used it in a neurological context to refer to the body schema's representation in the mind (Rizzuto 1990). He also used the term to refer to the psychological "representation" of instinct as affects and ideation. (This concept is discussed in Chapter 8.)

49. Putnam 1988.
50. Descartes 1628, p. 158.
51. Berlin 1956, p. 48.
52. Taylor 1989.
53. I have described this history in greater detail in *Object Love and Reality* (Modell 1968).
54. James 1890, p. 196.
55. Sandler and Rosenblatt 1962.
56. Beebe and Lachmann 1988.
57. James 1904, p. 173.
58. Ibid., p. 178.
59. Myers 1986.
60. James 1902, p. 135.
61. Winnicott 1974.
62. Perry 1935, p. 324.
63. Myers 1986.
64. Freud 1923, p. 13.
65. James 1890a.
66. Ibid., p. 299.
67. Ibid., p. 294.
68. Ibid., p. 315.
69. Ibid., p. 310.
70. James 1890, p. 336.
71. Ibid., p. 339.
72. Myers 1986, p. 362.
73. Modell 1990.
74. Edelman 1987.
75. Glauber 1963, p. 85.
76. Federn 1952.

77. For a fuller discussion of Federn's theoretical contributions, see Bergmann 1963.

78. Ibid., p. 97.

79. Jacobson 1954.

80. Anzieu 1989.

2.   *Private and Public Selves*

1. Kohut 1982.

2. Kohut 1980, p. 452.

3. Edelman 1989.

4. Goldstein 1940, p. 142.

5. Freud 1923, p. 26.

6. Schilder 1950.

7. Hull 1990, p. 64.

8. Greenacre 1958.

9. Edelman 1987.

10. Edelman 1989.

11. Edelman is of course referring to the biological self and not to personhood.

12. Edelman 1989, p. 93, emphasis added. In a highly speculative essay tracing the evolution of consciousness, Julian Jaynes suggests, on the basis of archeological evidence, that there was a time in man's history when the consciousness of self did not exist. In the absence of discrete selves, the cohesive social structure of early city-states may have been based upon the sharing of auditory hallucinatory experiences attributed to the gods. See Jaynes 1976.

13. Edelman 1989, p. 93. See Chapter 8 below for further discussion of the concept of value.

14. Ibid., p. 99, emphasis added.

15. Ibid., p. 98.

16. Ibid., p. 102.

17. The concept of reentry is difficult to convey to the reader who is not familiar with Edelman's more complete theory of Neural Darwinism. The interested reader should refer to Edelman 1987, 1989, 1992. "Reentry" refers to the brain's built-in coordinated signaling be-

tween anatomically separated structures that map both perceptual and conceptual categories. In a very broad sense, one can speculate that reentry generates the experience of coherence which is an essential aspect of the self. In *Bright Air, Brilliant Fire* (Edelman 1992), Edelman discusses the evolutionary significance of reentry. Edelman suggests that in the course of evolution, reentrant circuits appeared as a new component in neuroanatomy. These circuits that map and coordinate value-laden memories with incoming perceptual categories provide the organism with a certain degree of autonomy and freedom. Edelman further suggests that reentry processes contribute to the coherence of images of ongoing events.

18. Ibid., p. 158.
19. Sacks 1990.
20. Stern 1985.
21. White 1963.
22. The French philosopher Emmanuel Levinas states that "enjoyment is the very pulsation of the I" and that "one becomes a subject of being not by assuming being but in enjoying happiness." See Levinas 1969, pp. 113 and 119.
23. Brazelton 1980.
24. White 1963, p. 35.
25. Sander 1983.
26. Soref, unpublished.
27. Stern (1985, p. 229) proposed that we divide self experiences into a "social self," a "private self," and a "disavowed self."
28. Demos and Kaplan 1986.
29. Spitz 1957.
30. Fairbairn 1952.
31. Winnicott 1954.
32. Bibring 1953, p. 40.
33. Winnicott 1958, p. 33.
34. Stoller 1975.
35. Winnicott 1949.
36. Winnicott 1971, p. 65.
37. Ibid., p. 71.
38. Winnicott 1960, p. 51.

39. A similar idea is to be found in Bion's theory of the container and the contained (Bion 1970).

40. Winnicott 1960a, p. 150.

41. Ibid., p. 148.

42. Winnicott 1960, p. 46.

43. Ibid.

44. Winnicott 1967, p. 118.

45. Winnicott 1963, p. 189.

46. Rorty 1986, p. 9.

47. Ricoeur 1986.

48. Kohut 1984.

49. Kohut 1980, p. 454, emphasis added; ibid., p. 452.

50. Wolf 1988, pp. 11, 15.

51. Kohut 1977, pp. 171–219.

52. Kohut 1984.

53. Menaker 1982; Loewald 1984; Modell 1986.

54. See Modell 1984 for a discussion of Vico in relation to psychoanalytic knowledge.

55. Ricoeur 1986 and Toulmin 1986 have described self psychology and its roots in phenomenology. For a discussion of Kohut's philosophic position from within self psychology, see Goldberg 1988.

56. Nissim-Sabat 1989.

57. Husserl 1931, pp. 181, 198.

58. Kohut 1984, p. 32.

59. Bowlby 1969 and 1973.

60. I discuss this issue in a critical essay on self psychology (Modell 1986).

61. Kohut 1984, p. 197.

62. Taylor 1989, p. 137.

63. MacIntyre 1984, p. 172.

64. For an extraordinary synthesis of the origins of the idea of self in Western civilization, see Taylor 1989.

65. Ibid.

66. Ibid., p. 136.

67. Mead 1982, p. 148.

68. For further discussion, see Pfeutze 1961.

69. Feher-Gurewich 1989.

70. Mead 1982, p. 148.
71. Pfeutze 1961.
72. Sullivan 1950.
73. Ibid., p. 329.
74. Riesman, Glazer, and Denny 1950.
75. I describe a changing ecology of the neurosis in my essay "A Sociological Postscript," in *Psychoanalysis in a New Context* (Modell 1984).
76. Trilling 1971.
77. Ibid., p. 20.
78. Ariès 1962, p. 398.
79. Goffman 1956.
80. Collins 1985.
81. Goffman 1956, p. 2.
82. Taylor 1989.
83. Goffman 1956, p. 8.

3. The Private Self in Public Space

1. Lakoff 1987.
2. Ibid., p. 281.
3. Though the need for private space is a basic human requirement, one might object that physical privacy is a fairly modern development in Western culture (Ariès 1962). One wonders, then, how individuals found private space when there was little physical privacy. It is plausible that religious practice offered individuals the possibility of being alone with their thoughts, of becoming aware of their soul, their innermost self. One might then also ask: What happens to private space in countries like contemporary China or India, where the population density affords little chance for physical privacy? V. S. Naipaul, in *India, A Million Mutinies Now* (1991), provides a possible answer with regard to that particular subcontinent. He found that people, in the absence of physical privacy, became virtually obsessed with maintaining their individuality through a passionate devotion to personal interpretations of religious or political beliefs. That is to say, the personal self was kept alive through passionate interests. The

social history of literal private space is presented in the series *A History of Private Life* (Ariès and Duby 1987–1991).

4. James 1890, p. 291.

5. Freud 1930, p. 83.

6. Winnicott 1963, p. 77.

7. Fairbairn (1952), in his descriptive account of the schizoid personality, described the schizoid's fear of being drained when in the company of others.

8. Ibid., p. 16.

9. See *Psychoanalysis in a New Context* (Modell 1986).

10. The analyst is trained to listen for the metacommunications that accompany the spoken words. When the patient is reclining on the couch, both participants are deprived of the clues afforded by facial expressions. This situation is not unlike that of the blind person who relies on hearing. See, for example, John Hull's sensitive autobiographical account of the experience of becoming totally blind after years of normal sight. Hull describes how he became attuned to unintended nuances of the voice. "The capacity of the voice to reveal the self is truly amazing. Is the voice intelligent? Is it colorful? Is there light and shade? Is it gentle, amusing, varied? On the other hand is the voice lazy? Is it sloppy, careless? Is it flat, drab, monotonous?" (Hull 1990, p. 24).

11. Modell 1985a.

12. Laing 1960.

13. I have described this in Modell 1975a and 1980.

14. See Modell 1986, 1990.

15. Hull 1990, p. 217.

16. Modell 1990.

17. Modell 1976.

18. Modell 1990.

19. Freud 1933, p. 80.

20. Lacan 1977, p. 128.

21. Winnicott 1958, p. 34.

22. There are observational data to support the premise that affective experience forms the earliest core of the self (Emde 1988).

23. Laing 1960.
24. Stern 1985; Beebe and Lachmann 1987.
25. Bion 1970.
26. Summarized in Stern 1985.
27. Bakhtin 1984, p. 96, emphasis added.
28. Cited in MacIntyre 1981.
29. Sacks 1990.
30. I describe this process in Modell 1968 and 1984a.
31. Freud 1930, p. 130.
32. Faimberg 1988.
33. Murdoch 1985.
34. MacIntyre, discussing social roles in classical Greece, observed that in Sophocles' tragedies the hero is what society takes him or her to be. "But he or she is not only what society takes them to be, he or she both *belongs to a place in the social order and transcends it*" (MacIntyre 1981, p. 141). The hero is able to transcend his or her socially bestowed identity by encountering and acknowledging conflict. The key lies in transcending one's assigned role through the mastery of conflict.
35. Modell 1984b.
36. Maslow 1972, p. 42.
37. Anthony and Cohler 1987, p. 181.
38. Robinson 1985.
39. Shengold 1989.
40. Bergman 1988.
41. Hull 1990, p. 184.
42. Toulmin 1986.
43. Murdoch 1986.

4. The Dialectic of Self and Other

1. Atwood and Stolorow (1984) approach the psychology of intersubjectivity from a different philosophical direction. They see the roots of intersubjectivity in phenomenology and existential philosophy. This is consistent with their adherence to Kohut's self psychology.

2. Irving Singer has presented a panoramic exploration of the nature of love in Western culture, from Plato to the modern world (Singer 1984, 1984b, 1987).

3. For an appreciation of Hegel's relevance for contemporary psychology and psychoanalysis, see Hundert 1989; Benjamin 1990; and Kirschner 1991.

4. Hegel 1807.

5. Solomon 1985.

6. Winnicott 1971.

7. Taylor 1975, p. 159.

8. Hegel 1807, p. 234.

9. Ibid., p. 234, emphasis added.

10. Taylor 1975, p. 158.

11. Hegel 1807, p. 232.

12. Forrester 1990.

13. Modell 1984a, p. 131.

14. Hegel 1807, p. 234.

15. Winnicott 1971.

16. For an illustration of "reaching the point of maximum destructiveness," see Margaret Little's account of her analysis with Winnicott (Little 1985).

17. I have illustrated this point in a clinical vignette (Modell 1985).

18. Freud 1911, p. 220.

19. Freud 1915a, p. 134.

20. Ibid., p. 119.

21. Mahler, Pine, and Bergman 1975.

22. Ibid., p. 7.

23. Stern 1985.

24. Ibid., p. 21.

25. Trevarthen 1989.

26. Beebe and Lachmann 1987.

27. Winnicott 1971, p. 2.

28. Bateson 1972.

29. It is probable that psychoanalytic treatment could not proceed in the absence of a multileveled self. For it is absolutely essential that both

therapist and patient be able to shift back and forth from ordinary life to the frame that encloses the therapeutic process. For a detailed account, see *Other Times, Other Realities* (Modell 1990).

30. James 1890a, p. 287.

31. Ibid., p. 295.

32. This suggests that the much maligned concept of psychic energy may yet have some heuristic value if taken as a metaphor.

33. Freud 1925, p. 237.

34. Freud 1915a, p. 136, emphasis added.

35. Fairbairn 1952.

36. Klein 1948.

37. Freud 1933, p. 133.

38. Winnicott 1947.

39. Chasseguet-Smirgel 1985; Rycroft 1955.

40. Trivers 1985.

41. Modell 1991a.

42. Singer (1987), in his analysis of Freud as a philosopher of love, observed that overestimation is a defining characteristic of Freud's concept of love.

43. In this paper on narcissism, Freud did not differentiate between the terms "ego ideal" and "ideal ego." To complicate matters further, he would later, with the development of structural theory, subsume the ego ideal into the superego. Many authors have seen the usefulness of maintaining a distinction between the ego ideal and the superego (Novey 1955; Chasseguet-Smirgel 1985; Sandler 1963; Hanley 1984). I feel quite certain that the superego should be differentiated from the ego ideal for many reasons. Freud considered the superego a phylogenetic structure, analogous to other bodily organs that are the result of an evolutionary process. Although Freud recognized that there may be individual variations in the formation of the superego, and that it is modified in the development of the individual, he emphasized its inexorable impersonal quality. In contrast, the ego ideal reflects a personal morality. This subject will be examined further in Chapter 8.

44. Freud 1914, p. 94.

45. Balint 1959.

46. Kohut 1977, p. 185.
47. Ibid., p. 172.
48. Kohut 1984.
49. Modell 1990.
50. Modell 1988, 1988a.
51. Modell 1984.
52. Winnicott 1971.
53. Milner 1957.
54. Levinas 1961.
55. Ibid., p. 37.
56. Ibid., p. 45.
57. Bakhtin 1984.
58. Ibid., p. 22.
59. See also *Object Love and Reality* (Modell 1968), where this theme is developed further.
60. Freud 1907.
61. This formed the central thesis of my earlier book *Other Times, Other Realities* (Modell 1990).

5.   *The Generative Aspects of the Self*

1. Winnicott 1958, p. 34.
2. Ibid., p. 36.
3. Schafer (1968) refers to "presences" of indeterminate location as "primary process presences." Sandler (1990) connects the experience of an internal presence to internalized objects.
4. Freud 1917a, p. 399.
5. Langer 1967, pp. 88, 210.
6. Ariès 1962, p. 398: "The historians taught us that the King was never left alone. But in fact until the end of the seventeenth century, nobody was ever left alone. The density of social life made isolation virtually impossible, and people who managed to shut themselves up in a room for some time were regarded as exceptional characters."
7. James 1902, p. 42.
8. Ibid., emphasis added.
9. Klein 1963.

10. Fromm-Reichmann 1990.
11. Adler and Buie 1979.
12. Sacks 1973.
13. Quoted in Storr 1988, p. 36.
14. Thoreau 1854, p. 46.
15. Fromm-Reichmann 1990.
16. Monk 1990.
17. Ibid., p. 93.
18. Ibid., p. 94, emphasis added.
19. Ibid.
20. Ibid., p. 114.
21. Ibid., p. 141.
22. Ibid., p. 116.
23. Ibid., p. 319.
24. Eagle 1981.
25. James 1902, p. 162.
26. Murdoch 1985, p. 42.
27. Storr 1988.
28. Ibid., p. xii.
29. Kohut 1984, p. 52.
30. James 1902, p. 386.
31. Ibid., p. 107.
32. Ibid., p. 61.
33. Robert Graves 1948.
34. Ibid., p. 25.
35. Ibid., p. 24.
36. Richard Graves 1990.
37. Ibid., p. 54.
38. Ibid., p. 78.
39. Richardson 1991.
40. Ibid., p. 245, emphasis added.
41. Modell 1975.
42. Modell 1984, 1990.
43. For further discussion, see Modell 1990.
44. Winnicott 1971, p. 89.
45. I reported one such clinical vignette in Modell 1988.

46. Modell 1990a.
47. Gordon 1988.
48. Ibid., p. 62.
49. Ibid., p. 100.
50. Gay 1988, p. 56.
51. Ibid., p. 56.
52. Ibid., p. 57.
53. Ibid., p. 60.

6. *Process and Experience*

1. Rorty 1986, p. 4.
2. Applegarth 1989.
3. Sandler and Joffe 1969, p. 82.
4. Ibid.
5. Fairbairn 1952.
6. Ibid., p. 62.
7. Edelman 1989; Modell 1990.
8. For an extensive review of the concept of projective identification, see Sandler 1987; Tansey and Burke 1989.
9. Edelman's theory of Neural Darwinism assumes that memory is not isomorphic with past events but consists of categories that map such events (Edelman 1987, 1989). I have applied this theory to the understanding of projective identifications (Modell 1990).
10. In certain forms of severe depression characterized by psychomotor retardation, there is a loss of the sense of the efficacy of the self. Consequently the self ceases to be a creator of meaning, and there is a massive sense of emptiness and of absence of meaning. This goes far beyond the familiar loss of self esteem that accompanies depressive disorders.
11. Kristeva (1989) has discussed this loss of meaning in severe depressions and has suggested that speech has an activating as well as an inhibitory effect on neurobiological processes.
12. Kernberg (1976) believes that splitting of the self is a fundamental aspect of the psychopathology of borderline states.
13. Winnicott 1974.

14. Ibid., p. 91.
15. Grotstein 1990, 1990a, 1991.
16. Green 1986.
17. Freud 1917b, p. 248.
18. Shevrin 1988.
19. Marcel 1988.
20. Ibid.
21. Bollas 1987.
22. Freud 1895.
23. For a view that takes issue with Freud's commitment to neurophysiology, see Grossman 1992.
24. Solomon 1974.
25. Freud stated (1915, p. 174): "But every attempt to go on from there to discover a localization of mental processes, every endeavor to think of ideas as stored up in nerve-cells and of excitations as travelling along nerve-fibers, has miscarried completely." But then he adds: "Our psychical topography has *for the present* nothing to do with anatomy."
26. Pribram and Gill, 1976.
27. Klein 1976.
28. Gill 1976.
29. Klein 1976, p. 62.
30. For a more extensive summary of Freud's equivocation concerning neurophysiology, see Pribram and Gill 1976.
31. Freud 1915.
32. Ibid.
33. For a current discussion, see Putnam 1988.
34. Morton Reiser (1990) has extensively reviewed Freud's theory of dreams and dreaming in light of the contributions of contemporary neurobiology. Reiser's orientation with regard to the mind/brain problem differs from my own in several respects. In an earlier publication (1984), he viewed the mind and the brain as separate but analogous domains. He came to recognize, however, that with regard to affects there can be only one domain, as evidenced in the special psychophysiological conditions that exist during REM sleep. Reiser now accepts the widespread assumption that the brain is analogous to a

Turing machine, a computer employed in the processing of information in an algorithmic fashion. Edelman's theory of Neural Darwinism directly challenges this assumption.

35. Freud 1915a.
36. Ibid., p. 167, emphasis added.
37. Searle 1989.
38. Ibid., p. 201, emphasis added on "possible."
39. Edelman 1989, p. 92.
40. Ibid., p. 102.
41. Ibid., p. 152.
42. That evolution is a prediction of the past is a comment attributed to Ernst Mayr.
43. Freud 1900, p. 169. For further commentary and elaboration on this dream, see Palombo 1988 and Reiser 1990.
44. Edelman 1989.
45. In *Other Times, Other Realities* (Modell 1990), I describe how trauma foreshortens current time: only memories of the past select what is salient in the present, thus constricting current perceptions.
46. Masson 1985, p. 207.
47. Winnicott 1971a, p. 65.
48. Putnam 1988.
49. Quine 1987.
50. Beres and Joseph 1970.
51. Hull 1990.
52. Ibid., p. 144.

7. Private Meaning and the Agency of the Self

1. Nozick (1981, p. 574) lists no fewer than eight modes of meaning. His last definition is the one I have adopted here: "Meaning as personal significance, importance and value."
2. For further discussion, see Modell 1990.
3. Modell 1984.
4. Johnson 1987; Lakoff 1987.
5. Lakoff 1987, pp. 380–480.
6. This is a central thesis of *Other Times, Other Realities* (Modell 1990).

7. Millikan 1984, p. 150.

8. Rommetveit 1985.

9. Ibid., p. 187.

10. Modell 1991a.

11. For further discussion of this, see "Experiencing Time," in *Other Times, Other Realities* (Modell 1990).

12. Ibid.

13. Freud 1917c, p. 285.

14. Rorty 1986.

15. Freud 1933, p. 80.

16. Freud 1923, p. 23.

17. Freud 1933, p. 73.

18. Freud 1923, p. 30.

19. Modell 1990, p. 71.

20. Stern 1985; Beebe and Lachmann 1988.

21. Lakoff 1987, p. 310.

22. Freud 1920.

23. Winnicott (1960, p. 47): "Under favorable conditions the infant establishes a continuity of existence and then begins to develop the sophistication which makes it possible for impingements to be gathered into the area of omnipotence."

24. Freud identified this child as his grandson (Freud 1900, p. 461n).

25. Lacan (1977) gave a different interpretation. He emphasized the binary linguistic elements in the child's game and called this dynamic the "fort/da." In his view, the child's game represented the child's entry into the symbolic order of language. This entry into language Lacan saw as paradoxical—as both a submission and an extension of the self. It was a submission to the rules of language, which Lacan called "The Name of the Father."

26. Winnicott 1974, p. 91, emphasis added.

27. Rorty (1986, p. 5) says that Freud populated inner space with analogues of persons—internally coherent clusters of beliefs and desires. Each of these quasi persons, is, in the Freudian picture, part of a single unified *causal* network. Knowledge of all these persons is necessary to predict and control a human being's behavior (and in particu-

lar his or her "irrational" behavior), but at any given time only one of these persons will be available to introspection.

28. Edelman 1989, p. 287.

29. Freud (1926, p. 93): "[Anxiety] is reproduced as an affective state in accordance with an already existing mnemic image. If we go further and enquire into the origin of that anxiety—and of affects in general—we shall be leaving the realm of pure psychology and entering the borderland of physiology. Affective states have become incorporated in the mind as precipitates of primeval traumatic experiences, and when a similar situation occurs they are revived like mnemic symbols."

30. Modell 1991.

31. Van der Kolk and van der Hart 1989.

32. Ferenczi 1933.

33. Modell 1991a.

34. In Modell 1985, I presented a clinical vignette to illustrate this point.

35. See *Other Times, Other Realities* (Modell 1990), especially chs. 2, 3, and 4.

36. Freud's letter to Fliess of 6 December 1896 (Masson 1985, p. 207). See also Chapter 6, above.

37. Laplanche 1991.

38. Taylor 1989, p. 480.

39. Iris Murdoch (1985, p. 25), in a discussion of personal morality, observes that a person may make a specialized, individual use of a concept: "he derives the concept from his surroundings but takes it away into his privacy."

40. Bakhtin 1984, p. 22.

41. Levinas 1961.

42. Geertz 1983.

43. Schafer 1992.

44. Ibid., p. 156.

45. Ricoeur 1984, p. 52.

46. Ibid., p. 54.

47. For further discussion of this point, see *Other Times, Other Realities* (Modell 1990).

48. Bruner 1990.
49. Ibid., p. 170n42. Bruner is citing *A History of Private Life,* ed. Philippe Ariès and Georges Duby, trans. Arthur Goldhammer, 5 vols. (Cambridge, Mass.: Harvard University Press, 1987–1991).
50. Kakar 1985.

8.   *The Emergent Motives of the Self*

1. Kuhn 1962.
2. Kohut 1982, p. 401.
3. Edelman 1992.
4. Bowie 1991, p. 6.
5. Schafer 1976, p. 89.
6. Schafer 1983.
7. Schafer 1992.
8. Sullaway 1983.
9. Grossman 1992.
10. Parisi (1987) has argued that Freud was not committed to evolutionary biology because he rejected Darwinian evolution in favor of a Lamarckian theory of the inheritance of acquired characteristics. The fact that Freud was a neo-Lamarckian does not alter his belief that instinct could be explained phylogenetically. Gould (1977, p. 96) spells out how Lamarck thought about the origin of instincts: "Instincts are the unconscious remembrance of things learned. [These things are] impressed so indelibly into memory, that the germ cells themselves are affected and pass the trait to future generations."
11. Freud 1915, p. 124.
12. Gould 1977.
13. Freud 1915.
14. Freud (1923a, p. 258): "Though psycho-analysis endeavors as a rule to develop its theories as independently as possible from those of other sciences, it is nevertheless obliged to seek a basis for the theory of instincts in biology."
15. Freud 1923a, p. 258.
16. Freud 1920, p. 60.

17. Strachey consistently translated *Trieb* as "instinct" and explained his reasons for doing so (Standard Edition, vol. 14, p. 111).

18. Laplanche and Pontalis 1973, p. 214.

19. Freud 1915, p. 121.

20. Freud 1923a, p. 255, emphasis added.

21. Loewald 1988.

22. For a discussion of the concept of regression, see Modell 1990.

23. Abraham 1927.

24. Some of the following discussion is taken from Modell 1990b.

25. Lorenz 1935.

26. Hinde 1970; Mayr 1982; Trivers 1985.

27. Wilson 1975.

28. Mayr 1988. Lakoff (1987) also discusses the error of thinking of categories as an essentialist concept.

29. See Lakoff's discussion of essentialism as applied to categories (Lakoff 1986, p. 161).

30. Bateson 1972.

31. Freud (1915, p. 122) described instincts as having a somatic source (such as the endocrines), an aim (that which produces satisfaction by removing the stimulation from the source), and an object ("the thing which or through which the instinct is able to achieve its aim").

32. Bowlby 1969, 1973.

33. Winnicott 1956.

34. For further discussion of this point, see Modell 1975.

35. When Winnicott (1958, pp. 33–34) introduced the concept of ego relatedness, he wondered—perhaps out of a need to be consistent with Freud's instinct concept—whether we shouldn't consider the concept of *ego orgasm!*

36. Winnicott 1963, p. 181.

37. Loewald 1980, p. 127.

38. Ibid., p. 130.

39. Loewald 1980, 1988.

40. Greenberg 1991.

41. Solomon 1974.

42. Freud 1915a, p. 207.

43. Solomon 1974.

44. See, for example, the discussions in Solomon 1974; Draenos 1982; and Grossman 1992.

45. Edelson 1988.

46. Pantin (1968) has said that there is a fundamental contrast between *restricted* and *unrestricted* sciences. The biological sciences are unrestricted in that the biologist must be prepared to follow their problems into any other science whatsoever, whereas physical sciences are restricted in the sense that they do not require the investigator to traverse the other sciences.

47. Holzman and Aronson 1992.

48. The biological assumptions of psychoanalysis have been extensively reviewed in Slavin and Kriegman 1992.

49. See Gedo and Goldberg 1973; and, more recently, *The Biology of Clinical Encounters* (Gedo 1991).

50. Levin 1991.

51. Reiser, 1984, 1990.

52. Putnam 1988.

53. For further discussion of this important point, see Mayr 1988 (as it applies to biological concepts) and Lakoff 1987 (with regard to linguistic and cognitive concepts).

54. Mayr 1963, p. 5.

55. Edelman 1992.

56. Edelman, 1987, 1989, 1992.

57. Lorenz 1965, p. 44, emphasis added.

58. Lichtenberg (1989) has described motivational systems based on similar biological considerations. He outlines five motivational systems: (1) the need for psychic regulation of physiological requirements; (2) the need for attachment; (3) the need for exploration and assertion; (4) the need to react adversely through anger and withdrawal; (5) the need for sensual enjoyment and sexual excitement.

59. Goldstein 1940.

60. Lichtenstein (1961) attributed human identity to a "nonprocreative human sexuality." Psychoanalysts have long recognized the emergent motivations of the self. But instinct theory could not provide the necessary concepts to describe these emergent motivations, inasmuch

as there was no choice but to attribute motives to either the sexual or the aggressive instinct.

61. Winnicott 1963a, p. 77.
62. Trivers 1985. For an extensive discussion of the implications of Trivers' kinship theory for psychoanalysis, see Slavin and Kriegman 1992.
63. Modell 1991a.
64. Bruner (1990) has emphasized the use of narrative as a means not so much of maintaining the coherence of the private self but of "adjudicating" the differences between private and public construals of reality.
65. Singer 1992.
66. Hull 1990, p. 192.
67. Winnicott 1960.
68. The evolutionary significance of self actualization and its influence on mind and art have been brilliantly portrayed by Susanne Langer in *Mind: An Essay on Human Feeling,* vol. 1 (Langer 1967).
69. Loewald (1988) has valiantly attempted to explain this higher emergent property of "sublimation" in the context of Freud's libido theory.
70. Hinde 1970, p. 427.
71. Tomkins 1988.
72. Emde (1988) also discussed the significance of genetically fixed aspects of personality in child development in the context of Freud's "Analysis Terminable and Interminable."

References

Abraham, Karl. 1927. *Selected Papers on Psycho-Analysis.* Rpt. 1948. London: Hogarth Press.

Adler, Gerald, and Dan Buie. 1979. "Aloneness and borderline psychopathology: The possible relevance of child developmental issues." *International Journal of Psycho-analysis* 60 (1): 83–96.

Anthony, James, and Bertram Cohler. 1987. *The Invulnerable Child.* New York: Guilford Press.

Anzieu, Didier. 1989. *The Skin Ego.* Trans. Chris Turner. New Haven: Yale University Press.

Applegarth, Adrienne. 1989. "On Structures." *Journal of the American Psychoanalytic Association* 37 (4): 1097–1107.

Ariès, Philippe. 1962. *Centuries of Childhood.* New York: Knopf.

———— and Georges Duby, eds. 1987–1991. *A History of Private Life.* Trans. Arthur Goldhammer. 5 vols. Cambridge, Mass.: Harvard University Press.

Bakhtin, Mikhail. 1984. *The Dialogical Principle.* Trans. Wlad Godzich. Minneapolis: University of Minnesota Press.

Balint, Michael. 1959. *Thrills and Regressions.* New York: International Universities Press.

Bateson, Gregory. 1972. "Metalogue: What is an instinct?" In *Steps Towards an Ecology of Mind.* New York: Ballantine Books.

Beebe, Beatrice, and Frank Lachmann. 1988. "The contributions of mother-infant mutual influence to the origins of self- and object representations." *Psychoanalytic Psychology* 5 (4): 305–337.

Beres, David, and Edward Joseph. 1970. "The concept of mental representation in psychoanalysis." *International Journal of Psycho-analysis* 51 (1): 1–10.

Bergman, Ingmar. 1988. *The Magic Lantern.* Trans. Joan Tate. New York: Viking.

Bergmann, Martin. 1963. "The place of Paul Federn's ego psychology in psychoanalytic metapsychology." *Journal of the American Psychoanalytic Association* 11 (1): 97–116.

Berlin, Isaiah. 1956. "Locke." In *The Age of Enlightenment.* New York: Mentor.

Bibring, Edward. 1953. "The mechanism of depression." In *Affective Disorders: Psychoanalytic Contributions to Their Study,* ed. Phyllis Greenacre. New York: International Universities Press.

Bion, W. R. 1970. *Attention and Interpretation.* New York: Basic Books.

Bollas, Christopher. 1987. *The Shadow of the Object.* New York: Columbia University Press.

Bowie, Malcolm. 1991. *Lacan.* Cambridge, Mass.: Harvard University Press.

Bowlby, John. 1969. *Attachment.* New York: Basic Books.

——— 1973. *Attachment and Loss.* New York: Basic Books.

——— 1990. *Darwin.* New York: W. W. Norton.

Brazelton, T. Berry. 1980. "Neonatal assessment." In George Pollock and Stanley Greenspan, eds., *The Course of Life,* vol. 1. Washington: U.S. Department of Health and Human Services.

Bruner, Jerome. 1990. *Acts of Meaning.* Cambridge, Mass.: Harvard University Press.

Chasseguet-Smirgel, Janine. 1985. *The Ego Ideal.* New York: W. W. Norton.

Collins, Randall. 1985. *Three Sociological Traditions.* New York: Oxford University Press.

Dawson, Michael. 1985. "W. R. D. Fairbairn: Relating his work to his life." Diss., Harvard University.

Demos, Virginia, and Samuel Kaplan. 1986. "Motivation and affect reconsidered: Affect biographies of two infants." *Psychoanalysis and Contemporary Thought* 9 (2): 147–221.

Descartes, René. 1628. *Philosophical Works of Descartes.* Vol. 1. Rpt. 1955. Trans. Elizabeth Haldane and G. R. T. Ross. New York: Dover.

Draenos, Stan. 1982. *Freud's Odyssey.* New Haven: Yale University Press.

Eagle, Morris. 1981. "Interests as object relations." *Psychoanalysis and Contemporary Thought* (4): 527–565.

Edelman, Gerald. 1987. *Neural Darwinism: The Theory of Neuronal Group Selection*. New York: Basic Books.

——— 1989. *The Remembered Present: A Biological Theory of Consciousness*. New York: Basic Books.

——— 1992. *Bright Air, Brilliant Fire*. New York: Basic Books.

Edelson, Marshall. 1988. *Psychoanalysis: A Theory in Crisis*. Chicago: University of Chicago Press.

Emde, Robert. 1988. "Development terminable and interminable, I. Innate and motivational factors from infancy." *International Journal of Psycho-analysis* 69 (1): 23–42.

Erikson, Erik. 1959. *Psychological Issues,* vol. 1: *Identity and the Life Cycle*. New York: International Universities Press.

Faimberg, Haydé. 1988. "The telescoping of generations." *Contemporary Psychoanalysis* 24 (1): 99–118.

Fairbairn, W. R. D. 1952. *Psychoanalytic Studies of the Personality*. London: Tavistock.

Federn, Paul. 1952. *Ego Psychology and the Psychoses*. New York: Basic Books.

Feher-Gurewich, Judith. 1989. "Becoming a subject in the social world: The paradoxes of human desire." Diss., Brandeis University.

Ferenczi, Sándor. 1933. "Confusion of tongues between adults and the child." In *Final Contributions to the Problems and Methods of Psychoanalysis*. 1955. New York: Brunner/Mazel.

Fine, Reuben. 1990. *The History of Psychoanalysis*. New York: Continuum.

Forrester, John. 1990. *The Seductions of Psychoanalysis*. Cambridge: Cambridge University Press.

Foucault, Michel. 1990. *The History of Sexuality*. 1978. New York: Vintage.

Freud, Sigmund. 1895. "Project for a scientific psychology." In *The Standard Edition of the Complete Psychological Works,* 24 vols. Trans. James Strachey. London: Hogarth, 1953–. Hereafter abbreviated "*S.E.*"

——— 1900. "The interpretation of dreams." In *S.E.,* vol. 4.

——— 1900a. "The interpretation of dreams (second part)." In *S.E.,* vol. 5.

——— 1907. "Delusions and dreams in Jensen's Gravida." In *S.E.,* vol. 9.

———— 1911. "Formulations on the two principles of mental functioning." In *S.E.*, vol. 12.

———— 1914. "On narcissism: An introduction." In *S.E.*, vol. 14.

———— 1915. "Instincts and their vicissitudes." In *S.E.*, vol. 14.

———— 1915a. "The unconscious." In *S.E.*, vol. 14.

———— 1917. "Mourning and melancholia." In *S.E.*, vol. 14.

———— 1917a. "Introductory lectures on psychoanalysis (part III)." In *S.E.*, vol. 16.

———— 1920. "Beyond the pleasure principle." In *S.E.*, vol. 18.

———— 1921. "Group psychology and the analysis of the ego." In *S.E.*, vol. 18.

———— 1923. "The ego and the id." In *S.E.*, vol. 19.

———— 1923a. "Two encyclopaedia articles." In *S.E.*, vol. 18.

———— 1925. "Negation." In *S.E.*, vol. 19.

———— 1926. "Inhibitions, symptoms and anxiety." In *S.E.*, vol. 20.

———— 1930. "Civilization and its discontents." In *S.E.*, vol. 21.

———— 1933. "New introductory lectures on psychoanalysis." In *S.E.*, vol. 22.

———— 1937. "Analysis terminable and interminable." In *S.E.*, vol. 23.

———— 1940. "An outline of psychoanalysis." In *S.E.*, vol. 23.

———— 1987. *A Phylogenetic Fantasy.* Cambridge, Mass.: Harvard University Press.

Fromm-Reichmann, Frieda. 1990. "Loneliness." *Contemporary Psychoanalysis* 26 (2): 305–330.

Gay, Peter. 1988. *Freud: A Life for Our Time.* New York: W. W. Norton.

Gedo, John. 1991. *The Biology of Clinical Encounters.* Hillsdale, N.J.: Analytic Press.

———— and Arnold Goldberg. 1973. *Models of the Mind.* Chicago: University of Chicago Press.

Geertz, Clifford. 1983. *Local Knowledge.* New York: Basic Books.

Gill, Merton. 1976. "Metapsychology is not psychology." *Psychological Issues* 9 (4): 71–105. In Merton Gill, ed., *Psychology versus Metapsychology.* New York: International Universities Press.

Gilman, Sander. 1991. "Reading Freud in English: Problems, paradoxes and a solution." *International Review of Psychoanalysis* 18 (3): 331–344.

Glauber, Peter. 1963. "Federn's annotation of Freud's theory of anxiety." *Journal of the American Psychoanalytic Association* 11 (1): 84–96.

Goffman, Erving. 1956. *The Presentation of Self in Everyday Life.* Monograph no. 2. Edinburgh: University of Edinburgh Social Science Research Center.

Goldstein, Kurt. 1940. *Human Nature.* Cambridge, Mass.: Harvard University Press.

Gordon, Lyndall. 1988. *Eliot's New Life.* New York: Farrar, Straus and Giroux.

Gould, Stephen. 1977. *Ontogeny and Phylogeny.* Cambridge, Mass.: Harvard University Press.

Graves, Richard. 1990. *Robert Graves.* New York: Viking.

Graves, Robert. 1948. *The White Goddess.* Rpt. 1966. New York: Farrar, Straus and Giroux.

Green, André. 1986. *On Private Madness.* Madison, Conn.: International Universities Press.

Greenacre, Phyllis. 1958. "Early physical determinants of the development of the sense of identity." *Journal of the American Psychoanalytic Association* 6 (4): 612–627.

Greenberg, Jay. 1991. *Oedipus and Beyond.* Cambridge, Mass.: Harvard University Press.

——— and Stephen Mitchell. 1983. *Object Relation in Psychoanalytic Theory.* Cambridge, Mass.: Harvard University Press.

Grossman, William. 1982. "The self as fantasy: Fantasy as theory." *Journal of the American Psychoanalytic Association* 30 (4): 919–937.

——— 1992. "Hierarchies, boundaries and representation in the Freudian model of mental organization." *Journal of the American Psychoanalytic Association* 40 (1): 27–62.

——— and Bennett Simon. 1969. "Anthropomorphism: Motive, meaning, and causality in psychoanalytic theory." *Psychoanalytic Study of the Child* 24: 78–111.

Grotstein, James. 1990. "Nothingness, meaninglessness, chaos and the 'black hole.'" *Contemporary Psychoanalysis* 26 (2): 257–290.

——— 1990a. "Nothingness, meaninglessness, chaos and the 'black hole': Part 2." *Contemporary Psychoanalysis* 26 (3): 377–407.

————— 1991. "Nothingness, meaninglessness, chaos and the 'black hole': Part 3." *Contemporary Psychoanalysis* 27 (1): 1–33.

Hartmann, Heinz. 1939. *Ego Psychology and the Problem of Adaptation.* Rpt. 1958. Trans. David Rappaport. New York: International Universities Press.

————— 1950. "Comments on the psychoanalytic theory of the ego." *Psychoanalytic Study of the Child* 5: 74–96.

————— 1956. "Notes on the reality principle." *Psychoanalytic Study of the Child* 11: 31–53.

—————, Ernst Kris, and Rudolph Loewenstein. 1946. "Comments on the formation of psychic structure." *Psychoanalytic Study of the Child* 2: 11–38.

Hegel, G. W. F. 1807. *The Phenomenology of Mind.* Rpt. 1967. Trans. J. B. Baillie. New York: Harper Torchbooks.

Hinde, Robert. 1970. *Animal Behavior.* New York: McGraw-Hill.

Holzman, Philip, and Gerald Aronson. 1992. "Psychoanalysis and its neighboring sciences: Paradigms and opportunities." *Journal of the American Psychoanalytic Association* 40 (1): 63–88.

Hughes, Judith. 1989. *Reshaping the Psychoanalytic Domain.* Berkeley: University of California Press.

Hull, John. 1990. *Touching the Rock.* New York: Pantheon.

Hume, David. 1739. *Treatise on Human Nature.* Rpt. 1961. New York: Doubleday.

Hundert, Edward. 1989. *Philosophy, Psychiatry and Neuroscience.* Oxford: Clarendon Press.

Husserl, Edmund. 1931. "Consciousness and natural reality." In William Barrett and Henry Aiken, eds., *Philosophy in the Twentieth Century.* 1962. New York: Random House.

Jacobson, Edith. 1954. "Federn's contribution to ego psychology and psychoses." *Journal of the American Psychoanalytic Association* 2 (3): 519–525.

James, William. 1890. *The Principles of Psychology.* Vol. 1. 1950. New York: Dover.

————— 1890a. *The Principles of Psychology.* Vol. 2. 1950. New York: Dover.

————— 1902. *The Varieties of Religious Experience.* 1958. New York: Mentor.

———— 1904. "Does 'consciousness' exist?" In *The Writings of William James,* ed. John McDermott. Chicago: University of Chicago Press.

Jaynes, Julian. 1976. *The Origin of Consciousness in the Breakdown of the Bicameral Mind.* Boston: Houghton Mifflin.

Johnson, Mark. 1987. *The Body in the Mind.* Chicago: University of Chicago Press.

Kakar, Sudhir. 1985. "Psychoanalysis and non-Western cultures." *International Review of Psychoanalysis* 12 (4): 441–448.

Kernberg, Otto. 1976. *Object Relations Theory and Clinical Psychoanalysis.* New York: Jason Aronson.

———— 1982. "Self, ego, affects, drives." *Journal of the American Psychoanalytic Association* 30 (4): 893–917.

Klein, George. 1976. *Psycho-analytic Theory.* New York: International Universities Press.

Klein, Melanie. 1948. *Contributions to Psycho-Analysis.* London: Hogarth.

———— 1963. *Our Adult World.* New York: Basic Books.

Kohut, Heinz. 1977. *The Restoration of the Self.* New York: International Universities Press.

———— 1980. "Two letters." In Arnold Goldberg, ed., *Advances in Self Psychology.* New York: International Universities Press.

———— 1982. "Introspection, empathy and the semi-circle of mental health." *International Journal of Psycho-analysis* 63 (4): 396–407.

———— 1984. *How Does Analysis Cure?* Chicago: University of Chicago Press.

Kristeva, Julia. 1989. *Black Sun.* New York: Columbia University Press.

Kuhn, Thomas. 1962. *The Structure of Scientific Revolutions.* Chicago: University of Chicago Press.

Lacan, Jacques. 1977. *Ecrits.* Trans. Alan Sheridan. New York: W. W. Norton.

Laing, R. D. 1960. *The Divided Self.* London: Tavistock.

Lakoff, George. 1987. *Women, Fire, and Dangerous Things.* Chicago: University of Chicago Press.

Langer, Susanne. 1967. *Mind: An Essay on Human Feeling.* Vol. 1. Baltimore: Johns Hopkins University Press.

Laplanche, Jean. 1991. "Specificity of terminological problems in the translation of Freud." *International Review of Psychoanalysis* 18 (3): 401–406.

———— and J.-B. Pontalis. 1973. *The Language of Psycho-Analysis.* Trans. D. Nicholson-Smith. New York: W. W. Norton.

Lear, Jonathan. 1990. *Love and Its Place in Nature.* New York: Farrar, Straus and Giroux.

Levin, Fred. 1991. *Mapping the Mind.* Hillsdale, N.J.: Analytic Press.

Levinas, Emmanuel. 1961. *Totality and Infinity.* Pittsburgh: Duquesne University Press.

Lichtenberg, Joseph. 1989. *Psychoanalysis and Motivation.* Hillsdale, N.J.: Analytic Press.

Lichtenstein, Heinz. 1961. "Identity and sexuality: A study of their interrelationship in man." *Journal of the American Psychoanalytic Association* (9): 179–260.

———— 1963. "The dilemma of human identity: Notes on self-transformation, self-objectivation, and metamorphosis." *Journal of the American Psychoanalytic Association* 11: 173–223.

Little, Margaret. 1985. "Winnicott working." *Free Associations* 3: 9–42.

Loewald, Hans. 1980. "Instinct theory, object relations and psychic structure formation." In *Papers on Psychoanalysis.* New Haven: Yale University Press.

———— 1984. "Book review: The selected papers of Margaret Mahler." *Journal of the American Psychoanalytic Association* 32 (1): 165–175.

———— 1988. *Sublimation: Inquiries into Theoretical Psychoanalysis.* New Haven: Yale University Press.

Lorenz, Konrad. 1935. "Companionship in bird life." Trans. Claire Schiller. In Claire Schiller, ed., *Instinctive Behavior.* 1957. New York: International Universities Press.

———— 1965. *Evolution and the Modification of Behavior.* Chicago: University of Chicago Press.

MacIntyre, Alasdair. 1981. *After Virtue.* Notre Dame, Ind.: University of Notre Dame Press.

Mahler, Margaret, and Fred Pine. 1975. *The Psychological Birth of the Human Infant.* New York: Basic Books.

Marcel, Anthony. 1988. "Electrophysiology and meaning in cognitive science." In Mardi Horowitz, ed. *Psychodynamics and Cognition*. Chicago: University of Chicago Press.

Maslow, Abraham. 1972. *The Farther Reaches of Human Nature*. New York: Penguin.

Masson, Jeffrey, ed. and trans. 1985. *The Complete Letters of Sigmund Freud to Wilhelm Fliess*. Cambridge, Mass.: Harvard University Press.

Mayr, Ernst. 1963. *Animal Species and Evolution*. Cambridge, Mass.: Harvard University Press.

——— 1982. *The Growth of Biological Thought*. Cambridge, Mass.: Harvard University Press.

——— 1988. *Toward a New Philosophy of Biology*. Cambridge, Mass.: Harvard University Press.

McIntosh, Donald. 1986. "The ego and the self in the thought of Sigmund Freud." *International Journal of Psycho-analysis* 67 (4): 429–448.

Mead, George Herbert. 1982. *The Individual and the Social Self*. Ed. David Miller. Chicago: University of Chicago Press.

Menaker, Esther. 1982. *Otto Rank*. New York: Columbia University Press.

Millikan, Ruth. 1984. *Language, Thought, and Other Biological Categories*. Cambridge, Mass.: MIT Press.

Milner, Marion. 1957. *On Not Being Able to Paint*. New York: International Universities Press.

Modell, Arnold. 1968. *Object Love and Reality*. New York: International Universities Press.

——— 1975. "The ego and the id: Fifty years later." *International Journal of Psycho-analysis* 56 (1): 57–68.

——— 1975a. "A narcissistic defense against affects and the illusion of self-sufficiency." *International Journal of Psycho-analysis* 56 (3): 275–282.

——— 1976. "'The holding environment' and the therapeutic action of psychoanalysis." *Journal of the American Psychoanalytic Association* 24 (2): 285–307.

——— 1980. "Affects and their non-communication." *International Journal of Psycho-analysis* 61 (2): 259–267.

——— 1984. "Contexts and complementarity." In *Psychoanalysis in a New Context.* New York: International Universities Press.

——— 1984a. *Psychoanalysis in a New Context.* New York: International Universities Press.

——— 1984b. "On having the right to a life." In *Psychoanalysis in a New Context.* New York: International Universities Press.

——— 1985. "Object relations theory." In Arnold Rothstein, ed., *Models of the Mind.* New York: International Universities Press.

——— 1985a. "Self preservation and the preservation of the self." *Annual of Psychoanalysis* 12/13: 69–86.

——— 1986. "The missing elements in Kohut's cure." *Psychoanalytic Inquiry* 6 (3): 367–385.

——— 1988. "On the protection and safety of the therapeutic setting." In Arnold Rothstein, ed., *How Does Treatment Help?* Madison, Conn.: International Universities Press.

——— 1988a. "The persistence of transitional relatedness." In Paul Horton, Herbert Gewitz, and Karole Kreutter, eds., *The Solace Paradigm.* Madison, Conn.: International Universities Press.

——— 1990. *Other Times, Other Realities: Toward a Theory of Psychoanalytic Treatment.* Cambridge, Mass.: Harvard University Press.

——— 1990a. "The roots of creativity and the use of the object." In Peter Giovacchini, ed., *Tactics and Techniques in Psychoanalytic Psychotherapy,* vol. 3. Northvale, N.J.: Aronson.

——— 1990b. "Some notes on object relations, 'classical' theory, and the problem of instincts (drives)." *Psychoanalytic Inquiry* 10 (2): 182–196.

——— 1991. "Review of Hans Loewald's *Sublimation: Inquiries into Theoretical Psychoanalysis.*" *Psychoanalytic Quarterly* 60 (3): 467–470.

——— 1991a. "A confusion of tongues, or whose reality is it?" *Psychoanalytic Quarterly* 60 (2): 227–244.

Monk, Ray. 1990. *Ludwig Wittgenstein.* New York: Free Press.

Murdoch, Iris. 1985. *The Sovereignty of Good.* London: Routledge and Kegan Paul.

Myers, Gerald. 1986. *William James.* New Haven, Conn.: Yale University Press.

Nagel, Thomas. 1974. "Freud's anthropomorphism." In Richard Wollheim, ed., *Freud*. New York: Anchor Books.

Naipaul, V. S. 1990. *India: A Million Mutinies Now*. New York: Viking.

Nissim-Sabat, Marilyn. 1989. "Kohut and Husserl." In Douglas Detrick and Susan Detrick, eds., *Self Psychology: Comparisons and Contrasts*. Hillside, N.J.: Analytic Press.

Nozick, Robert. 1981. *Philosophical Explanations*. Cambridge, Mass.: Harvard University Press.

Ornston, Darius. 1982. "Strachey's influence." *International Journal of Psycho-analysis* 63 (4): 409–426.

——— 1985. "The invention of 'cathexis' and Strachey's strategy." *International Review of Psychoanalysis* 12 (4): 391–400.

——— 1985a. "Freud's conception is different from Strachey's." *Journal of the American Psychoanalytic Association* 33 (2): 379–412.

Palombo, Stanley. 1988. "Day residue, screen memory in Freud's botanical monograph dream." *Journal of the American Psychoanalytic Association* 36 (4): 881–904.

Pantin, C. F. A. 1968. *The Relations between the Sciences*. Cambridge: Cambridge University Press.

Parisi, Thomas. 1987. "Why Freud failed: Some implications for neurophysiology and sociobiology." *American Psychologist* 42 (3): 235–245.

Perry, Ralph Barton. 1935. *The Thought and Character of William James*. Vol. 1. Boston: Little, Brown.

Pfeutze, Paul. 1961. *Self, Society, Existence*. New York: Harper Torchbooks.

Pribram, Karl, and Merton Gill. 1976. *Freud's "Project" Re-assessed*. New York: Basic Books.

Putnam, Hilary. 1988. *Representation and Reality*. Cambridge, Mass.: MIT Press.

Quine, W. V. 1987. *Quiddities*. Cambridge, Mass.: Harvard University Press.

Reiser, Morton. 1984. *Mind, Brain, Body*. New York: Basic Books.

——— 1990. *Memory in Mind and Brain*. New York: Basic Books.

Richardson, John. 1991. *A Life of Picasso*. New York: Random House.

Ricoeur, Paul. 1984. *Time and Narrative*. Chicago: University of Chicago Press.

———— 1986. "The self in psychoanalysis and in phenomenological philosophy." *Psychoanalytic Inquiry* 6 (3): 437–458.

Riesman, David, Nathan Glazer, and Reuel Denney. 1950. *The Lonely Crowd*. New York: Doubleday Anchor.

Rizzuto, Ana-Maria. 1990. "The origins of Freud's concept of object representation: 'On aphasia.'" *International Journal of Psychoanalysis* 71 (2): 241–248.

Robinson, David. 1985. *Chaplin*. New York: McGraw-Hill.

Rommetveit, Ragnar. 1985. "Language acquisition as increasing linguistic structuring of experience and symbolic behavior control." In James Wertsch, ed., *Culture, Communication and Cognition: Vygotskian Perspectives*. Cambridge: Cambridge University Press.

Rorty, Richard. 1986. "Freud and moral reflection." In Joseph Smith and William Kerrigan, eds., *Pragmatism's Freud: The Moral Disposition of Psychoanalysis*. Baltimore: Johns Hopkins University Press.

Rycroft, Charles. 1955. "Two notes on idealization, illusion and disillusion as normal and abnormal psychological processes." *International Journal of Psycho-analysis* 36 (2): 81–87.

Sacks, Oliver. 1973. *Awakenings*. 1990. New York: Harper Perennial.

———— 1990. "Neurology and the soul." *New York Review of Books* 18 (November 22): 44–50.

Sander, Louis. 1983. "Polarity, paradox and the organizing process of development." In Justin Call and Robert Tyson, eds., *Frontiers of Infant Psychiatry*. New York: Basic Books.

Sandler, Joseph. 1987. "The concept of projective identification." In Joseph Sandler, ed., *Projection, Identification, Projective Identification*. Madison, Conn.: International Universities Press.

———— 1990. "On internal object relations." *Journal of the American Psychoanalytic Association* 38 (4): 859–880.

———— and Bernard Rosenblatt. 1962. "The concept of the representational world." *Psychoanalytic Study of the Child* 17: 128–145.

Sandler, Joseph, and Walter Joffe. 1969. "Towards a basic psychoanalytic model." *International Journal of Psycho-analysis* 50 (1): 79–90.

Schafer, Roy. 1968. *Aspects of Internalization*. New York: International Universities Press.

——— 1976. *A New Language for Psychoanalysis*. New Haven: Yale University Press.

——— 1983. *The Analytic Attitude*. New York: Basic Books.

——— 1992. *Retelling a Life*. New York: Basic Books.

Schilder, Paul. 1950. *The Image and Appearance of the Human Body*. New York: International Universities Press.

Searle, John. 1989. "Consciousness, unconsciousness, and intentionality." *Philosophical Topics* 17 (1): 193–209.

Shengold, Leonard. 1989. *Soul Murder*. New Haven: Yale University Press.

Shevrin, Howard. 1988. "Unconscious conflict: A convergent psychodynamic and electrophysiological approach." In Mardi Horowitz, ed., *Psychodynamics and Cognition*. Chicago: University of Chicago Press.

Singer, Irving. 1992. *Meaning in Life*. New York: Free Press.

Slavin, Malcolm, and Daniel Kriegman. 1992. *The Adaptive Design of the Human Psyche*. New York: Guilford Press.

Solomon, Robert. 1974. "Freud's neurological theory of mind." In Richard Wollheim, ed., *Freud: A Collection of Critical Essays*. New York: Doubleday Anchor.

——— 1985. *In the Spirit of Hegel*. New York: Oxford University Press.

Soref, Alice. Unpublished. "The self, in and out of relatedness."

Spitz, René. 1957. *No and Yes*. New York: International Universities Press.

Spruiell, Van. 1981. "The self and the ego." *Psychoanalytic Quarterly* 50 (3): 319–344.

Stern, Daniel. 1985. *The Interpersonal World of the Infant*. New York: Basic Books.

Stoller, Robert. 1975. *Perversion: The Erotic Form of Hatred*. Washington: American Psychiatric Press.

Storr, Anthony. 1988. *Solitude: A Return to the Self*. New York: Ballantine.

Sullivan, Harry. 1950. "The illusion of personal individuality." *Psychiatry* 13: 317–332.

Sulloway, Frank. 1979. *Freud: Biologist of the Mind.* New York: Basic Books.

Sutherland, John. 1989. *Fairbairn's Journey into the Interior.* London: Free Association Books.

Tansey, Michael, and Walter Burke. 1989. *Understanding Countertransference.* Hillsdale, N.J.: Analytic Press.

Taylor, Charles. 1975. *Hegel.* Cambridge: Cambridge University Press.

———— 1989. *Sources of the Self.* Cambridge, Mass.: Harvard University Press.

Thoreau, Henry. 1854. *Walden.* Rpt. 1961. New York: Bramhall House.

Tomkins, Silvan. 1988. *Affect Imagery Consciousness.* Vol. 1. Rpt. 1962. New York: Springer.

Toulmin, Stephen. 1986. "Self psychology as a 'postmodern' science." *Psychoanalytic Inquiry* 6 (3): 459–477.

Trevarthen, Colwyn. 1989. "Intuitive emotions: Their changing role in communication beween mother and infant." In M. Ammaniti, ed., *Affetti: Natura e sviluppo delle relazione interpersonali.* Bari: Laterza.

Trilling, Lionel. 1971. *Sincerity and Authenticity.* Cambridge, Mass.: Harvard University Press.

Trivers, Robert. 1985. *Social Evolution.* Menlo Park, Calif.: Benjamin/Cummings.

Van der Kolk, Bessel, and Onno van der Hart. 1989. "Pierre Janet and the breakdown of adaptation in psychological trauma." *American Journal of Psychiatry* 146: 1330–1342.

———— 1991. "The intrusive past: The flexibility of memory and the engraving of trauma." *American Imago* 48 (4): 425–454.

White, Robert. 1963. "Ego and reality in psychoanalytic theory." In White, *Psychological Issues,* vol. 3. New York: International Universities Press.

Wilson, Edward. 1975. *Sociobiology.* Cambridge, Mass.: Harvard University Press.

Winnicott, Donald W. 1947. "Hate in the countertransference." In *Collected Papers.* 1958. New York: Basic Books.

———— 1949. "Mind and its relation to the psyche-soma." In *Collected Papers.* 1958. New York: Basic Books.

———— 1954. "Metapsychological and clinical aspects of regression within the psycho-analytical set-up." In *Collected Papers*. 1958. New York: Basic Books.

———— 1956. "Primary maternal preoccupation." In *Collected Papers*. 1958. New York: Basic Books.

———— 1958. "The capacity to be alone." In *The Maturational Processes and the Facilitating Environment*. 1965. New York: International Universities Press.

———— 1960. "The theory of the parent-infant relationship." In *The Maturational Processes and the Facilitating Environment*. 1965. New York: International Universities Press.

———— 1960a. "Ego distortions in terms of true and false self." In *The Maturational Processes and the Facilitating Environment*. 1965. New York: International Universities Press.

———— 1962. "Ego integration in child development." In *The Maturational Processes and the Facilitating Environment*. 1965. New York: International Universities Press.

———— 1963. "Communicating and not communicating leading to a study of certain opposites." In *The Maturational Processes and the Facilitating Environment*. 1965. New York: International Universities Press.

———— 1963a. "The capacity for concern." In *The Maturational Processes and the Facilitating Environment*. 1965. New York: International Universities Press.

———— 1967. "Mirror-role of mother and family in child development." In *Playing and Reality*. 1971. New York: Basic Books.

———— 1971. "The use of an object and relating through identifications." In *Playing and Reality*. New York: Basic Books.

———— 1971a. *Playing and Reality*. New York: Basic Books.

———— 1974. "Fear of breakdown." In Winnicott, *Psycho-analytic Explorations,* ed. Clare Winnicott, Ray Shepherd, and Madeleine Davis. 1989. Cambridge, Mass.: Harvard University Press.

Wolf, Ernest. 1988. *Treating the Self.* New York: Guilford Press.

Index

247